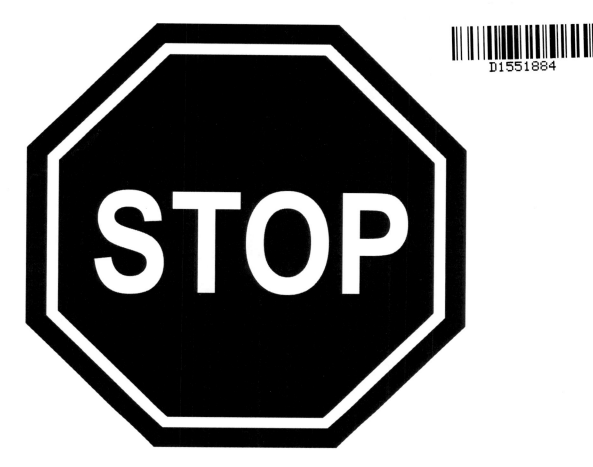

FREE Test Taking Tips DVD Offer

To help us better serve you, we have developed a Test Taking Tips DVD that we would like to give you for FREE. **This DVD covers world-class test taking tips that you can use to be even more successful when you are taking your test.**

All that we ask is that you email us your feedback about your study guide. Please let us know what you thought about it – whether that is good, bad or indifferent.

To get your **FREE Test Taking Tips DVD**, email freedvd@studyguideteam.com with "FREE DVD" in the subject line and the following information in the body of the email:

     a. The title of your study guide.

     b. Your product rating on a scale of 1-5, with 5 being the highest rating.

     c. Your feedback about the study guide. What did you think of it?

     d. Your full name and shipping address to send your free DVD.

If you have any questions or concerns, please don't hesitate to contact us at freedvd@studyguideteam.com.

Thanks again!

ACSM Certified Personal Trainer Study Guide

Exam Prep & Practice Test Questions
[5th Edition]

Joshua Rueda

Interested in buying more than 10 copies of our product? Contact us about bulk discounts:
bulkorders@studyguideteam.com

ISBN 13: 9781637754474
ISBN 10: 1637754477

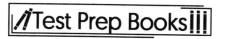

Table of Contents

Quick Overview

As you draw closer to taking your exam, effective preparation becomes more and more important. Thankfully, you have this study guide to help you get ready. Use this guide to help keep your studying on track and refer to it often.

This study guide contains several key sections that will help you be successful on your exam. The guide contains tips for what you should do the night before and the day of the test. Also included are test-taking tips. Knowing the right information is not always enough. Many well-prepared test takers struggle with exams. These tips will help equip you to accurately read, assess, and answer test questions.

A large part of the guide is devoted to showing you what content to expect on the exam and to helping you better understand that content. In this guide are practice test questions so that you can see how well you have grasped the content. Then, answer explanations are provided so that you can understand why you missed certain questions.

Don't try to cram the night before you take your exam. This is not a wise strategy for a few reasons. First, your retention of the information will be low. Your time would be better used by reviewing information you already know rather than trying to learn a lot of new information. Second, you will likely become stressed as you try to gain a large amount of knowledge in a short amount of time. Third, you will be depriving yourself of sleep. So be sure to go to bed at a reasonable time the night before. Being well-rested helps you focus and remain calm.

Be sure to eat a substantial breakfast the morning of the exam. If you are taking the exam in the afternoon, be sure to have a good lunch as well. Being hungry is distracting and can make it difficult to focus. You have hopefully spent lots of time preparing for the exam. Don't let an empty stomach get in the way of success!

When travelling to the testing center, leave earlier than needed. That way, you have a buffer in case you experience any delays. This will help you remain calm and will keep you from missing your appointment time at the testing center.

Be sure to pace yourself during the exam. Don't try to rush through the exam. There is no need to risk performing poorly on the exam just so you can leave the testing center early. Allow yourself to use all of the allotted time if needed.

Remain positive while taking the exam even if you feel like you are performing poorly. Thinking about the content you should have mastered will not help you perform better on the exam.

Once the exam is complete, take some time to relax. Even if you feel that you need to take the exam again, you will be well served by some down time before you begin studying again. It's often easier to convince yourself to study if you know that it will come with a reward!

Test-Taking Strategies

1. Predicting the Answer

When you feel confident in your preparation for a multiple-choice test, try predicting the answer before reading the answer choices. This is especially useful on questions that test objective factual knowledge. By predicting the answer before reading the available choices, you eliminate the possibility that you will be distracted or led astray by an incorrect answer choice. You will feel more confident in your selection if you read the question, predict the answer, and then find your prediction among the answer choices. After using this strategy, be sure to still read all of the answer choices carefully and completely. If you feel unprepared, you should not attempt to predict the answers. This would be a waste of time and an opportunity for your mind to wander in the wrong direction.

2. Reading the Whole Question

Too often, test takers scan a multiple-choice question, recognize a few familiar words, and immediately jump to the answer choices. Test authors are aware of this common impatience, and they will sometimes prey upon it. For instance, a test author might subtly turn the question into a negative, or he or she might redirect the focus of the question right at the end. The only way to avoid falling into these traps is to read the entirety of the question carefully before reading the answer choices.

3. Looking for Wrong Answers

Long and complicated multiple-choice questions can be intimidating. One way to simplify a difficult multiple-choice question is to eliminate all of the answer choices that are clearly wrong. In most sets of answers, there will be at least one selection that can be dismissed right away. If the test is administered on paper, the test taker could draw a line through it to indicate that it may be ignored; otherwise, the test taker will have to perform this operation mentally or on scratch paper. In either case, once the obviously incorrect answers have been eliminated, the remaining choices may be considered. Sometimes identifying the clearly wrong answers will give the test taker some information about the correct answer. For instance, if one of the remaining answer choices is a direct opposite of one of the eliminated answer choices, it may well be the correct answer. The opposite of obviously wrong is obviously right! Of course, this is not always the case. Some answers are obviously incorrect simply because they are irrelevant to the question being asked. Still, identifying and eliminating some incorrect answer choices is a good way to simplify a multiple-choice question.

4. Don't Overanalyze

Anxious test takers often overanalyze questions. When you are nervous, your brain will often run wild, causing you to make associations and discover clues that don't actually exist. If you feel that this may be a problem for you, do whatever you can to slow down during the test. Try taking a deep breath or counting to ten. As you read and consider the question, restrict yourself to the particular words used by the author. Avoid thought tangents about what the author *really* meant, or what he or she was *trying* to say. The only things that matter on a multiple-choice test are the words that are actually in the question. You must avoid reading too much into a multiple-choice question, or supposing that the writer meant something other than what he or she wrote.

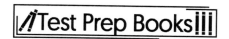

5. No Need for Panic

It is wise to learn as many strategies as possible before taking a multiple-choice test, but it is likely that you will come across a few questions for which you simply don't know the answer. In this situation, avoid panicking. Because most multiple-choice tests include dozens of questions, the relative value of a single wrong answer is small. As much as possible, you should compartmentalize each question on a multiple-choice test. In other words, you should not allow your feelings about one question to affect your success on the others. When you find a question that you either don't understand or don't know how to answer, just take a deep breath and do your best. Read the entire question slowly and carefully. Try rephrasing the question a couple of different ways. Then, read all of the answer choices carefully. After eliminating obviously wrong answers, make a selection and move on to the next question.

6. Confusing Answer Choices

When working on a difficult multiple-choice question, there may be a tendency to focus on the answer choices that are the easiest to understand. Many people, whether consciously or not, gravitate to the answer choices that require the least concentration, knowledge, and memory. This is a mistake. When you come across an answer choice that is confusing, you should give it extra attention. A question might be confusing because you do not know the subject matter to which it refers. If this is the case, don't eliminate the answer before you have affirmatively settled on another. When you come across an answer choice of this type, set it aside as you look at the remaining choices. If you can confidently assert that one of the other choices is correct, you can leave the confusing answer aside. Otherwise, you will need to take a moment to try to better understand the confusing answer choice. Rephrasing is one way to tease out the sense of a confusing answer choice.

7. Your First Instinct

Many people struggle with multiple-choice tests because they overthink the questions. If you have studied sufficiently for the test, you should be prepared to trust your first instinct once you have carefully and completely read the question and all of the answer choices. There is a great deal of research suggesting that the mind can come to the correct conclusion very quickly once it has obtained all of the relevant information. At times, it may seem to you as if your intuition is working faster even than your reasoning mind. This may in fact be true. The knowledge you obtain while studying may be retrieved from your subconscious before you have a chance to work out the associations that support it. Verify your instinct by working out the reasons that it should be trusted.

8. Key Words

Many test takers struggle with multiple-choice questions because they have poor reading comprehension skills. Quickly reading and understanding a multiple-choice question requires a mixture of skill and experience. To help with this, try jotting down a few key words and phrases on a piece of scrap paper. Doing this concentrates the process of reading and forces the mind to weigh the relative importance of the question's parts. In selecting words and phrases to write down, the test taker thinks about the question more deeply and carefully. This is especially true for multiple-choice questions that are preceded by a long prompt.

9. Subtle Negatives

One of the oldest tricks in the multiple-choice test writer's book is to subtly reverse the meaning of a question with a word like *not* or *except*. If you are not paying attention to each word in the question, you can easily be led astray by this trick. For instance, a common question format is, "Which of the following is...?" Obviously, if the question instead is, "Which of the following is not...?," then the answer will be quite different. Even worse, the test makers are aware of the potential for this mistake and will include one answer choice that would be correct if the question were not negated or reversed. A test taker who misses the reversal will find what he or she believes to be a correct answer and will be so confident that he or she will fail to reread the question and discover the original error. The only way to avoid this is to practice a wide variety of multiple-choice questions and to pay close attention to each and every word.

10. Reading Every Answer Choice

It may seem obvious, but you should always read every one of the answer choices! Too many test takers fall into the habit of scanning the question and assuming that they understand the question because they recognize a few key words. From there, they pick the first answer choice that answers the question they believe they have read. Test takers who read all of the answer choices might discover that one of the latter answer choices is actually *more* correct. Moreover, reading all of the answer choices can remind you of facts related to the question that can help you arrive at the correct answer. Sometimes, a misstatement or incorrect detail in one of the latter answer choices will trigger your memory of the subject and will enable you to find the right answer. Failing to read all of the answer choices is like not reading all of the items on a restaurant menu: you might miss out on the perfect choice.

11. Spot the Hedges

One of the keys to success on multiple-choice tests is paying close attention to every word. This is never truer than with words like almost, most, some, and sometimes. These words are called "hedges" because they indicate that a statement is not totally true or not true in every place and time. An absolute statement will contain no hedges, but in many subjects, the answers are not always straightforward or absolute. There are always exceptions to the rules in these subjects. For this reason, you should favor those multiple-choice questions that contain hedging language. The presence of qualifying words indicates that the author is taking special care with his or her words, which is certainly important when composing the right answer. After all, there are many ways to be wrong, but there is only one way to be right! For this reason, it is wise to avoid answers that are absolute when taking a multiple-choice test. An absolute answer is one that says things are either all one way or all another. They often include words like *every*, *always*, *best*, and *never*. If you are taking a multiple-choice test in a subject that doesn't lend itself to absolute answers, be on your guard if you see any of these words.

12. Long Answers

In many subject areas, the answers are not simple. As already mentioned, the right answer often requires hedges. Another common feature of the answers to a complex or subjective question are qualifying clauses, which are groups of words that subtly modify the meaning of the sentence. If the question or answer choice describes a rule to which there are exceptions or the subject matter is complicated, ambiguous, or confusing, the correct answer will require many words in order to be expressed clearly and accurately. In essence, you should not be deterred by answer choices that seem excessively long. Oftentimes, the author of the text will not be able to write the correct answer without

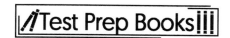

offering some qualifications and modifications. Your job is to read the answer choices thoroughly and completely and to select the one that most accurately and precisely answers the question.

13. Restating to Understand

Sometimes, a question on a multiple-choice test is difficult not because of what it asks but because of how it is written. If this is the case, restate the question or answer choice in different words. This process serves a couple of important purposes. First, it forces you to concentrate on the core of the question. In order to rephrase the question accurately, you have to understand it well. Rephrasing the question will concentrate your mind on the key words and ideas. Second, it will present the information to your mind in a fresh way. This process may trigger your memory and render some useful scrap of information picked up while studying.

14. True Statements

Sometimes an answer choice will be true in itself, but it does not answer the question. This is one of the main reasons why it is essential to read the question carefully and completely before proceeding to the answer choices. Too often, test takers skip ahead to the answer choices and look for true statements. Having found one of these, they are content to select it without reference to the question above. Obviously, this provides an easy way for test makers to play tricks. The savvy test taker will always read the entire question before turning to the answer choices. Then, having settled on a correct answer choice, he or she will refer to the original question and ensure that the selected answer is relevant. The mistake of choosing a correct-but-irrelevant answer choice is especially common on questions related to specific pieces of objective knowledge. A prepared test taker will have a wealth of factual knowledge at his or her disposal, and should not be careless in its application.

15. No Patterns

One of the more dangerous ideas that circulates about multiple-choice tests is that the correct answers tend to fall into patterns. These erroneous ideas range from a belief that B and C are the most common right answers, to the idea that an unprepared test-taker should answer "A-B-A-C-A-D-A-B-A." It cannot be emphasized enough that pattern-seeking of this type is exactly the WRONG way to approach a multiple-choice test. To begin with, it is highly unlikely that the test maker will plot the correct answers according to some predetermined pattern. The questions are scrambled and delivered in a random order. Furthermore, even if the test maker was following a pattern in the assignation of correct answers, there is no reason why the test taker would know which pattern he or she was using. Any attempt to discern a pattern in the answer choices is a waste of time and a distraction from the real work of taking the test. A test taker would be much better served by extra preparation before the test than by reliance on a pattern in the answers.

FREE DVD OFFER

Don't forget that doing well on your exam includes both understanding the test content and understanding how to use what you know to do well on the test. We offer a completely FREE Test Taking Tips DVD that covers world class test taking tips that you can use to be even more successful when you are taking your test.

All that we ask is that you email us your feedback about your study guide. To get your **FREE Test Taking Tips DVD**, email freedvd@studyguideteam.com with "FREE DVD" in the subject line and the following information in the body of the email:

- The title of your study guide.
- Your product rating on a scale of 1-5, with 5 being the highest rating.
- Your feedback about the study guide. What did you think of it?
- Your full name and shipping address to send your free DVD.

Introduction to the ACSM CPT

Function of the Test

The American College of Sports Medicine (ACSM) Certified Personal Trainer (CPT) Exam is for individuals who wish to become certified in the area of professional fitness in order to provide clients of varying fitness levels with resources to lead healthier and fitter lives. Candidates for the CPT portion of the ACSM exam must be eighteen years or older, must have a high school diploma or equivalent, and must have CPR with AED certification.

In 2015, for the ACSM CPT Exam, there were 5,226 candidates with a pass rate of 54%. In 2014, 5,152 candidates received a pass rate of 55%. As of June 2015, there were 13,999 ACSM Certified Personal Trainers.

Test Administration

Pearson VUE administers this computer-based exam in over 5,000 locations throughout the world. The exam costs $299. For ACSM members, a discount voucher is available to those who email the ACSM Certification Department at certification@acsm.org with their member ID and the exam name. If a candidate fails a test, they are given a retest code, which is found in the Failed Score Reports. This code can be used to receive discounts on future exams. Candidates may retest fifteen days after each failed test until the candidate earns a passing score.

Test Format

The ACSM CPT exam is separated into four domains, each based on a Job Task Analysis (JTA) that explains what someone with an ACSM CPT certification does on a daily basis. The four domains are Initial Client Consultation and Assessment; Exercise Programming and Implementation; Exercise Leadership and Client Education; and Legal, Professional, Business and Marketing.

The exam will provide candidates with a calculator when needed. No other materials or equipment will be allowed in the examination area.

All exams include "unscored" questions used to determine whether or not they are to be used for future exams. The unscored questions will be scattered throughout the exam, but will not be counted in the final score. The ACSM CPT exam features 120 scored and 30 unscored multiple-choice questions within a 2 hour and 35-minute time limit. The following table depicts the different domains and their question percentages:

Domain	Domain Title	Percentage of Questions
Domain I	Initial Client Consultation and Assessment	25%
Domain II	Exercise Programming and Implementation	45%
Domain III	Exercise Leadership and Client Education	20%
Domain IV	Legal, Professional, Business and Marketing	10%

Scoring

Candidates will receive their score as soon as they complete the exam, which will be given on a 200-800 scale. A passing score is 550 or higher.

Study Prep Plan for the ACSM CPT

1 **Schedule -** Use one of our study schedules below or come up with one of your own.

2 **Relax -** Test anxiety can hurt even the best students. There are many ways to reduce stress. Find the one that works best for you.

3 **Execute -** Once you have a good plan in place, be sure to stick to it.

One Week Study Schedule		
	Day 1	Initial Client Consultation and Assessment
	Day 2	Exercise Programming and Implementation
	Day 3	Practice Questions
	Day 4	Exercise Leadership & Client Education
	Day 5	Legal & Professional Responsibilities
	Day 6	Practice Questions
	Day 7	Take Your Exam!

Two Week Study Schedule				
	Day 1	Test-Taking Strategies; Intro to the ACSM CPT	Day 8	Exercise Leadership & Client Education
	Day 2	Initial Client Consultation and Assessment	Day 9	Practice Questions
	Day 3	Practice Questions	Day 10	Review Answer Key and Explanations
	Day 4	Review Answer Key and Explanations	Day 11	Legal & Professional Responsibilities
	Day 5	Exercise Programming and Implementation	Day 12	Practice Questions
	Day 6	Practice Questions	Day 13	Review Answer Key and Explanations
	Day 7	Review Answer Key and Explanations	Day 14	Take Your Exam!

One Month Study Schedule

Day 1	Providing Instructions and Initial Documents to the Client in Order to Proceed to the Interview	Day 11	The Principles of Specificity and Program Progression	Day 21	Creating a Positive Exercise Experience to Optimize Adherence
Day 2	Health Behavior Modification Theories and Strategies to Determine Client Goals	Day 12	Benefits, Risks, and Contraindications for Cardiovascular Training Exercises	Day 22	Health Coaching Principles
Day 3	Educating Clients on Modifiable Risk Factors	Day 13	Effective Implementation of the Components of an Exercise Program	Day 23	Relationship Between Body Composition and Health
Day 4	Directions of Body Movements	Day 14	Using Repetition Maximum Test Results to Determine Resistance Training Loads	Day 24	Practice Questions
Day 5	Muscle Actions	Day 15	Appropriate Teaching Techniques to Demonstrate Exercises for Improving Range of Motion	Day 25	Review Answer Key and Explanations
Day 6	Muscle Terms	Day 16	Safely Demonstrating Various Resistance-Training Modalities	Day 26	Reputable Referral Sources
Day 7	Referral to a Physician	Day 17	Normal and Abnormal Responses to Exercise and Criteria for Termination of Exercise	Day 27	Initial Management of Various Complications
Day 8	Practice Questions	Day 18	Proper and Improper Form and Technique for Flexibility Exercises	Day 28	Practice Questions
Day 9	Review Answer Key and Explanations	Day 19	Practice Questions	Day 29	Review Answer Key and Explanations
Day 10	Risks and Benefits of Exercise Training and Programming for Healthy Populations	Day 20	Review Answer Key and Explanations	Day 30	Take Your Exam!

Initial Client Consultation and Assessment

Providing Instructions and Initial Documents to the Client in Order to Proceed to the Interview

Personal trainers are health and fitness professionals who use an individualized approach to assess, educate, train, and motivate clients. They help clients identify reasonable and measurable goals, then design safe and effective exercise programs to achieve those goals. Personal trainers have the responsibility of interviewing potential clients prior to beginning a program in order to gather pertinent information regarding health, lifestyle, and exercise readiness. They also follow a health appraisal process to screen clients for risk factors and symptoms associated with cardiovascular, metabolic, pulmonary, and orthopedic conditions. This pre-participation health appraisal process optimizes the safety of exercise testing and programming.

Components and Preparation for the Initial Client Consultation

The initial client consultation is the first scheduled meeting between the client and the personal trainer and is intended to assess compatibility between trainer and client, determine client goals, develop an appropriate exercise/training program, and establish the client-trainer agreement. There are several key components and preparatory steps that a personal trainer should have in place for a new client prior to beginning an assessment or engaging in the actual exercise program. This preparation sets the groundwork for safe exercise, a positive and compatible client-trainer relationship, mutually agreed upon goal development, and the setting of appropriate expectations for both the trainer and the client. Specific documentation should be completed and reviewed. There should be a thorough discussion and written agreement related to pricing, policies (e.g., cancellations and missed sessions), where and when sessions will take place, what equipment is needed/provided by each party, and whether medical clearance from a physician is needed prior to commencement of the exercise training program.

Necessary Paperwork to be Completed by Client Prior to Initial Client Interview

There are several required documents to be completed initially by the client in order to proceed to the interview. Each of these forms warrants an in-person discussion of the content of the forms during the initial client consultation.

The Informed Consent Form gives clients information about the procedures and processes of the exercise program. This form should include a detailed description of the planned exercise program, a confidentiality clause (keeping pertinent client information private or for intended parties only), risks and benefits associated with participation, responsibilities of the client, and documentation of acknowledgement and acceptance of the stated items in the form.

The Client Intake Form includes basic identifying demographic information about the client, including contact information, height/weight, goals, reasons for starting an exercise program or seeking personal training, and any concerns.

The Health/Medical Evaluation Form assesses the appropriateness of moderate and vigorous levels of exercise by identifying positive risk factors associated with coronary artery disease (CAD), existing diagnosed pathologies, past surgical history, medications, orthopedic conditions, and lifestyle management. This form is used to help stratify the level of risk for the patient and the suitability of exercise testing and programming.

The Client/Trainer Agreement Form reinforces that the personal trainer and client are under contract law. It is a written document signed by both parties describing the services, the involved parties and expectations of each, as well as a timeline of delivery, cost, and payment, including aspects such as the cancellation policy and contract termination.

The Physical Activity Readiness Questionnaire (PAR-Q) is a questionnaire of self-recall, referring to signs and symptoms experienced by the client as well as information referring to diagnosed conditions. The purpose of this form is to screen and identify clients that require additional medical screening prior to exercise participation, while not excluding those who should be safe to start a low-intensity exercise program without physician approval (due to the known inherent benefits of physical activity and their low-risk stratification).

The Medical Clearance Form is a form signed by the client's physician after his or her evaluation. If the PAR-Q or other health appraisal screening information reveals that the client requires medical referral and physician clearance (e.g., one or more questions have been answered "yes" on the PAR-Q, client is over the age of forty and has not participated in regular physical activity for a substantial period of time), then additional attention may be required.

Effective Communication

Communication between the client and personal trainer is necessary for a successful, positive working relationship. It is important to use the initial client consultation to establish effective communication and establish expectations for communication moving forward. Both parties should feel comfortable expressing their thoughts, needs, concerns, and questions. Both parties should feel respected, fully listened to, and clearly responded to. The personal trainer must operate with confidentiality during communication, sharing client information only with those for whom written consent has been obtained.

Utilizing Multi-Media Resources and/or In-Person Resources

Communication takes on several forms: verbal, non-verbal (eye contact, tone of voice, gestures), written (email, handouts, articles), and via multi-media (texting). In the increasingly technological society, there is greater reliance on multi-media resources for communication including email, phone, and text messaging. Establishing expectations for such resources, such as acceptable times of day to call or text, as well as a reasonable timeframe for a response, should be established so that involved parties are on the same page. Preferred methods of contact and communication should also be discussed and documented in the client-trainer agreement to assess trainer-client compatibility. For instance, if the client wishes to communicate in person, but the trainer relies heavily on email or text, both parties must discuss and see if a compromise or agreement can be established for effective communication.

Interviewing Client in Order to Gather and Provide Pertinent Information

The trainer builds rapport with the client during the interview process by using a patient-centered approach, empathy, and active listening—a process of trying to understand the underlying meaning in a client's words. This positive approach has been shown to lead to higher client satisfaction and compliance as well as a decrease in client concerns. Asking open-ended questions and repeating or

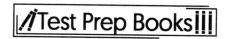

rephrasing responses in a clarifying manner is a form of active listening that builds a positive, trusting relationship. The trainer should encourage the client with verbal and non-verbal cues, make eye contact, look engaged, and not rush the client.

Components and Limitations of a Health/Medical History

The trainer should be aware that there are some limitations inherent to the health appraisal forms and screening tools. For instance, the PAR-Q is designed to determine the safety of exercise, but it does not necessarily identify any disease risks. The Informed Consent Form does not inherently relieve the personal trainer of the responsibility to perform in a competent manner under his or her scope of practice.

Sometimes these forms are augmented by the addition of a Release/Assumption of Risk Agreement. This form may be used for apparently healthy individuals with no known risk factors who want to begin an exercise program, but who decline to complete the necessary health appraisal forms. The Release/Assumption of Risk Agreement must identify the potential risks in participating in the exercise program and validate that the client understands these risks and voluntarily chooses to assume responsibility.

Lastly, the PAR-Q and certain medical history forms filled out by the client, rather than the physician, are based on client recall and self-support, leaving room for intentional or unintentional error. It is important to ensure that all forms including a clause are filled out as true and with full disclosure. They should also include the client's signature.

Use of Medical Clearance for Exercise Testing and Program Participation

A client must obtain medical clearance from a physician if he or she answers "yes" to any PAR-Q questions, experiences any signs or symptoms of cardiovascular or pulmonary disease, wants to participate in vigorous exercise (as a moderate risk stratification) or moderate exercise (with a high risk stratification). Additionally, previously inactive men over age forty and women over age fifty must obtain clearance.

Health Behavior Modification Theories and Strategies to Determine Client Goals

The Client Intake form, as well as the information gathered and discussed in the initial screening, should inform the personal trainer of the client's health and fitness goals, motivation, interests, and internal and environmental challenges. Goals should be discussed prior to any fitness testing and then be adjusted according to the physiological level of fitness, as well as to strengths and weaknesses garnered through the evaluation process. Training goals should address the greatest physiologic deficiencies, with each specific goal designed to address an area of weakness. Although clients may have other goals besides those for improving the most significant weaknesses, these should be prioritized because they may hold more of a personal weight to the client and yield higher levels of internal motivation.

Personal trainers should guide clients to make S.M.A.R.T goals: Specific, Measurable, Attainable, Realistic, and Timely. They may also need to give examples of what S.M.A.R.T goals look like. The importance of measurable and timely goals should not be understated, and progress towards goals should be periodically evaluated. Training programs should be designed with each client's goals in mind.

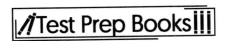

Orientation Procedures

An important component to include to ensure the safety of the exercise program is the client's complete understanding of the proper usage and location of the exercise equipment and facilities (bathrooms, towels, etc.) in the training facility. This education is a crucial role of the personal trainer, especially if there is an expectation of the client completing exercises at times other than scheduled sessions with the trainer. The personal trainer should keep in mind that there should be ongoing instruction throughout the program, including demonstrations of how to use and adjust equipment, how to maintain proper form, and the use of verbal cues, mirrors, and diagrams to assist instruction.

Obtaining a Health/Medical History, Medical Clearance and Informed Consent

The required documentation, such as the health/medical history and informed consent, are important in reducing liability for the trainer, optimizing the safety of the client, and creating the best customized training plan tailored to the specific client's needs and goals. These forms need to be completed, signed, and reviewed prior to participation. Health history forms inform the trainer of any cardiovascular risk factors that might be associated with physical activity. Obtaining proper medical clearance forms, when suggested and required, as well as signed informed consent forms helps protect the trainer from liability of any injury or discomfort experienced during and after sessions. The Client-Trainer Agreement Form communicates the policies and procedures, which (when discussed and agreed upon) position the trainer and client to have a successful professional relationship.

Reviewing and Analyzing Client Data to Formulate a Plan of Action and/or Conduct Physical Assessments

Client data collected at the initial interview is used to formulate a plan of action, which entails determining whether the client needs further medical evaluation and clearance, if fitness assessments can be scheduled, and if/when the exercise program can commence.

Risk Factors for Cardiovascular Disease

One of the main functions of the health appraisal process is to identify any potential risk for cardiovascular, pulmonary, and metabolic diseases for the client based on his or her current health. Personal trainers need to be familiar with the American College of Sports Medicine (ACSM) guidelines and risk factors for these diseases so they can appropriately stratify risk and, if needed, refer clients to medical specialists prior to engaging in an exercise program.

During a training session, a trainer must monitor the client for warning signs that require medical attention. Because some of these warnings can be dismissed as normal responses to exercise, it is imperative that a trainer be aware of specific symptoms that can result from cardiovascular distress. These may subside with a break that allows the heart rate to return to normal or the client to rehydrate. If signs persist, the trainer should recommend that the client consult a physician before re-initiating physical activity. If a client experiences any of the following symptoms while performing exercises, the trainer should immediately discontinue the workout, have the client rest and rehydrate, and, if necessary, seek medical assistance:

- Inappropriate changes to resting or exercise heart rate and blood pressure
- New-onset discomfort in chest, neck, shoulder, or arm
- Changes in the pattern of discomfort during rest or exercise

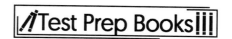

- Shortness of breath at rest or with light exertion
- Fainting or dizzy spells
- Intermittent claudication

While these symptoms are normal physical responses to vigorous exercise, trainers are responsible for recognizing when a client's symptoms indicate a serious complication. When in doubt, trainers should err on the side of caution, and refer the client to a physician for approval to continue with the exercise program; not only does this safeguard the client's health, but it also minimizes the risk of liability for the trainer.

Possible Symptoms of Chronic Cardiovascular, Metabolic, and/or Pulmonary Disease Chronic Cardiovascular Disease

Coronary artery disease (CAD) is associated with atherosclerosis: a progressive, degeneration of the endothelial lining and resultant hardening of the arterial walls. Arteries become less elastic and more narrow as plaque builds up inside, reducing blood-carrying capacity to the heart. While exercise can be protective against this disease process, if clients are already at increased disease risk, exercise may result in adverse coronary episodes due to the increased demand exercise places on an already compromised system.

Extensive research on CAD has identified positive risk factors: aspects of behavior, lifestyle, environmental exposures, or inherited traits that may increase the potential to acquire CAD. The greater the number of positive risk factors, the higher the risk of CAD and resultant issues with exercise. Positive risk factors include the following:

- History: family history of myocardial infarction, coronary revascularization, or sudden death in a first-degree relative before age fifty-five in males or sixty-five in females

- Cigarette smoking: current smoker or one who has quit in the previous six months

- Hypertension: taking antihypertensive medications or systolic blood pressure ≥ 140 mmHg or diastolic pressure ≥ 90 mmHg, confirmed by at least two separate measurements on different occasions

- Hypercholesterolemia: current use of lipid-lowering medications or total cholesterol > 200 mg/dL, LDL > 130 mg/dL or low HDL < 40 mg/dL

- Impaired fasting blood glucose: ≥ 100 mg/dL, confirmed by at least two separate measurements on different occasions

- Obesity: waist circumference of > 100cm (39 inches) or BMI ≥ 30 kg/m²

- Sedentary lifestyle: little to no exercise or failure to meet the U.S. Surgeon General's report's minimum physical activity recommendations of thirty minutes or more of moderate-intensity physical activity on most, if not all, days per week

Chronic Metabolic Disease

Diabetes mellitus is the primary metabolic disease of concern, affecting the body's ability to metabolize blood glucose. It is an independent risk factor for cardiovascular disease. There are two types of diabetes. In Type 1, there is a problem with insulin secretion, and patients are insulin dependent, requiring insulin injections for glucose metabolism. This is an autoimmune disease that typically presents early in life. In Type 2, patients produce enough insulin, but glycemic control is abnormal because the tissue does not respond adequately to the circulating insulin.

Symptoms indicative of possible metabolic disease include the following:

- Excess abdominal fat (men: waist circumference > 100 cm or 39 inches; women: waist circumference > 88 cm)
- Elevated triglyceride levels (> 150 mg/dL)
- Low HDL cholesterol (< 40 mg/dL)
- Elevated fasting glucose levels (> 100 mg/dL)
- Elevated blood pressure (> 140 mmHg systolic and > 90 mmHg diastolic)

Chronic Pulmonary Disease

Pulmonary diseases affect the ability of the respiratory system to transport oxygen to the tissues during exercise via the cardiovascular system, resulting in inadequate oxygen supply and reduced exercise capacity. Pulmonary disease symptoms mirror many of those for cardiovascular disease and include the following:

- Shortness of breath with mild exertion or even at rest
- Dizziness or syncope (fainting)
- Water retention or swelling in the ankles (edema) or calf cramping (intermittent claudication)
- Irregular heartbeat (palpitations) or rapid heartbeat (tachycardia) or known heart murmur
- Chest, neck, jaw, or arm pain due to limited blood flow (ischemia)
- The need to sit up to breathe easily (orthopnea)
- Unusual fatigue
- Breathlessness, especially at night (nocturnal dyspnea)

While not diagnostic in and of themselves, it is important that trainers be aware of these symptoms and refer clients to physicians for formal evaluations.

Medical Clearance, Exercise Testing, and Supervision Recommendations Based on Risk Stratification

A personal trainer should require medical clearance for clients who answer "yes" to any PAR-Q questions, experience any signs or symptoms of cardiovascular or pulmonary disease, or want to participate in vigorous exercise as a moderate risk stratification or moderate exercise with a high risk stratification.

Low risk: medical exam not needed prior to moderate or vigorous activity; physician supervision not necessary for maximal or submaximal testing

Medium risk: medical exam not needed prior to moderate activity, but recommended for vigorous activity; physician supervision not necessary for submaximal testing, but recommended for maximal testing

High risk: medical exam recommended prior to moderate or vigorous activity; physician supervision recommended for maximal or submaximal testing

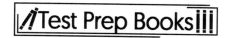

Educating Clients on Modifiable Risk Factors

The personal trainer should use ACSM guidelines to determine risk and stratify clients for their safety as well as to limit liability. When in doubt, it is better to err on the side of caution and obtain written physician clearance (prior to exercise participation) and include physician monitoring of exercise testing, particularly at maximal levels.

Certain cardiovascular disease risk factors are modifiable, and it is one of the trainer's responsibilities to help educate and support clients in engaging in lifestyle changes that lower disease risk. For example, clients who smoke should be educated about the dangers of smoking and directed to resources that help support quitting the habit. Engaging in regular exercise can help lower blood pressure and get clients active, rather than sedentary. Trainers should encourage healthy eating and provide information or referrals to professionals and resources that can further educate and improve a client's diet. Hypertension, hypocholesteremia, high triglycerides, and impaired blood glucose control can be reduced with a healthy diet.

Determining Appropriate Physical Assessments

The initial paperwork and interview yields information about the client's current health, physical fitness level, health/injury risk, and unique goals that can guide decisions about appropriate physical assessments. It is important to choose assessments that are safe, keeping in mind that depending on a client's stratification, physician supervision may be required and/or submaximal assessments should be used. Ideally, assessment selection should match goals or be something that can be monitored for improvements caused by targeted training during subsequent reassessments. For instance, if a client is going to be focusing primarily on a strength/resistance training program, using only an endurance assessment may not be the optimal choice.

Following Protocols During Fitness Assessment Administration

To ensure reliable data collection and scoring, tests should be conducted according to their established protocols and procedures, and in a logical order so that the client is safe and fatigue and testing error do not confound results.

Testing Equipment and Proper Use

To avoid errors in scores based on equipment malfunction or influence, all testing equipment should be assessed for proper function and be calibrated prior to use in testing. For example, prior to using a metabolic cart to measure expired gases, the cart should be calibrated by entering the environmental data (humidity, barometric pressure, temperature) as well as volume of expired air with the 3L calibration syringe. The use of some equipment also requires that certain preparation steps are followed to produce a valid response. For example, bioelectrical impedance machines to measure body fat are very sensitive to body water levels, so athletes should urinate before the test. In addition, prior to the test they cannot eat or drink for at least 30 minutes, exercise for at least 12 hours, drink alcohol for at least 48 hours, or consume caffeine.

Testing Procedures

Many tests have procedures for a warm-up and require proper rest between trials, but for those that do not have a warm-up built into the test, trainers should make sure that clients have performed a thorough warm-up of the metabolic and physiologic systems that will be used in the test. For example, if performing a 1RM bench press test, clients should warm up with light cardiovascular exercise to increase blood flow, heart rate, and muscle perfusion, then complete a few sets with increasing weight below max, to prepare the muscles for the test. Tests should also be recorded in a logical order with the most fatiguing assessments last.

Studies have found that strength scores are lower after cardiovascular endurance assessments, but not vice versa, so strength tests should be conducted prior to strenuous distance runs or 300-yard shuttle runs. If tests need to be repeated due to some sort of error, it is usually preferable to revisit them on another day so that any accumulated fatigue from the first attempt does not confound the subsequent re-take.

Evaluating Behavioral Readiness to and Developing Strategies to Optimize Exercise Adherence

The trans-theoretical model describes the client's process of getting ready to start exercise and consists of five stages:

- Pre-contemplation: Client is not intending to take action toward changing physical activity and is not considering becoming physically active.

- Contemplation: Client intends to increase physical activity within the next six months.

- Preparation: Client has developed a plan of action toward behavior change and will be making changes in the immediate future (next thirty days) and/or is inconsistently engaging in some amount of physical activity, but not at least thirty minutes of moderate-intensity activity for five or more days per week.

- Action: Client engages in at least thirty minutes of moderate-intensity activity for five or more days per week, but for less than six months.

- Maintenance: Client actively maintains changes made during the action stage, and new behaviors are established for six months or more; client is working to prevent relapse.

Behavioral Strategies to Enhance Exercise and Health Behavior Change

Feedback leads to the knowledge of results and is important in the progress toward goal achievement and evaluation of success or failure. Setting goals that are both appropriately difficult and personally motivating for the client will enhance commitment. Reinforcement can occur on a psychological level (influencing behavior and self-esteem or self-efficacy) and a neurobiological level (with the release of dopamine, which strengthens the synaptic pathways involved in learning a behavior).

The personal trainer should use feedback and positive reinforcement to enhance a client's self-efficacy and motivation towards health improvement. Positive, encouraging social support from peers, family, friends, or community can also enhance behavior change and goal achievement. Negative social support can cause feelings of doubt and inadequacy and lower self-esteem. The personal trainer should ask each client about the social support system he or she has and realize that many clients need the trainer to play a significant role of support.

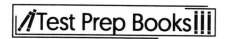

S.M.A.R.T. Goals

- Specific: clearly-defined (who, what, when, where, why, how)

- Measurable: a way to track progress and determine when the goal is achieved

- Attainable: make sure the goal is not out of reach

- Realistic: similar to attainable, but also making sure that goals are compatible with client's lifestyle, health, injury history, injuries, and time to train

- Timely: a specific date or timeframe for goals, which gives structure to the goal, helps it to be more measurable, and provides an appropriate sense of urgency, while still being practical and feasible in the allotted timeframe

Applications of Health Behavior Change Models

An understanding of behavioral change models will assist personal trainers in reinforcing positive behaviors and helping their clients avoid sabotaging progress towards behavioral goals. While there are many health behavior change models, several common ones are as follows:

- Health Belief Model: the perceived seriousness of a potential health problem as the main predictor of behavioral change

- Theory of Planned Behavior: client's level of motivation for behavioral change shaped by his or her attitudes, subjective norms, and perceived control—intention to engage in a behavior will ultimately result in that behavior

- Social Cognitive Theory: clients actively shaping their lives and learning by thinking, feeling, reflecting, and observing themselves in a social context

- Socio-Ecological Model: addresses relationships, behaviors (e.g., client's motivation to exercise) shaped by interpersonal relations, the surrounding environment, community, policy, and law

Setting Effective Client-Oriented Behavioral Goals

Goal setting is a strategic approach to address and implement positive behavioral changes through which progressive standards of success (short term goals) are set en route to a desired standard of achievement (long term goal). This systematic approach aids in a feeling of mastery, which increases motivation and commitment, leading to improved behavioral change. The personal trainer needs to take an individualized approach to the goal-setting process with clients, taking into account the person's interests and needs and not just relying on the results of testing to set goals.

Assessing Physical Fitness to Set Goals

A thorough assessment of physical fitness, including cardiorespiratory fitness, muscular strength, muscular endurance, flexibility, and anthropometric measures, will aid in establishing a baseline and setting appropriate goals. Goals should be diversified to include the various aspects of fitness, focusing on the greatest deficiencies and the client's interests. Recording baseline levels establishes a benchmark

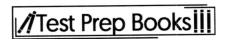

from which progress can be measured by conducting routine reassessments at regularly scheduled intervals.

Basic Structures of Bones, Skeletal Muscle, and Connective Tissue Bone

The skeleton is divided into the axial (skull, vertebrae, ribs, and sternum) and appendicular (shoulder girdles, arms, hips, legs) skeletons. There are two types of bone or osseous tissue. Compact (cortical) bone comprises 80 percent of bone mass and is made of dense, organized Haversian systems, which are arrangements of minerals, living bone cells, nerves, blood, and lymph vessels. Cancellous (spongy) bone, the other 20 percent of bone mass, lacks Haversian systems, is porous with trabeculae (lattice, branching arrangement), and has marrow and fat storage.

Skeletal Muscle
This muscle is voluntarily controlled by the nervous system and is elastic, extensible, and able to contract. It is striated, and cells have multiple nuclei.

Connective Tissue
The three major structures are tendons (attaching muscle to bone), ligaments (connecting bone to bone), and fascia (attaches, stabilizes, encloses, and separates muscles and other internal organs).

Basic Anatomy of Cardiovascular and Respiratory Systems

The heart has the smaller right and left atria on top of the larger right and left ventricles. A series of valves keeps blood flowing in the correct direction and prevents backflow to optimize cardiac efficiency: the bicuspid, tricuspid, pulmonary semilunar, and aortic semilunar valves.

The aorta is the main blood vessel branching off the top of the heart and sends blood to circulate through the body. The blood vessels, in order of decreasing size away from the heart, are arteries, arterioles, and capillaries. Towards the heart, from smallest to largest, are capillaries, venules, and veins.

Blood enters the (1) right atrium. When it contracts, blood passes through the (2) tricuspid valve into the (3) right ventricle. After filling, the right ventricle contracts, and the tricuspid valve closes, pushing blood through the (4) pulmonary semilunar valve into the (5) pulmonary arteries. These arteries, unlike all other arteries in the body, carry deoxygenated blood to the lungs, where blood travels through the (6) alveolar capillaries. Here, oxygen is absorbed and carbon dioxide is removed.

The newly-oxygenated blood is carried by the (7) pulmonary veins back to the (8) left atrium. Contraction of the left atrium moves blood through the (9) bicuspid valve into the (10) left ventricle (the largest heart chamber). When the bicuspid valve closes and the left ventricle contracts, blood is forced into the (11) aortic valve through the aorta and on to systemic circulation.

Heart Rate and Blood Pressure During Exercise
Both heart rate and systolic blood pressure increase linearly with exercise intensity.

Diastolic pressure may remain constant or decrease slightly over a bout of exercise, due to the reduced peripheral resistance that occurs during activity to facilitate oxygen delivery to muscles.

Age, fitness level, medications, temperature, hydration status, and body position can also affect heart rate.

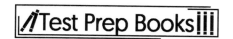

Directions of Body Movements

- Inferior: toward the feet
- Superior: toward the head
- Medial: toward the body's midline
- Lateral: away from the body's midline
- Supination: typically used to describe forearm or ankle motion, rotating up and inward
- Pronation: typically used to describe forearm or ankle motion, rotating down and outward
- Flexion: a reduction in joint angle by two segments of the body around one joint coming closer together
- Extension: an increase in joint angle by two segments of the body around one joint moving apart
- Adduction: movement toward the body's midline
- Abduction: movement away from the body's midline (typically out to the side)
- Hyperextension: movement beyond the normal extension range of a joint
- Rotation: turning to the right or left, often of the head or neck or ankles
- Circumduction: moving in a circular motion, a compound motion involving flexion, extension, abduction, and adduction into one movement
- Agonist: the primary muscle involved in a motion
- Antagonist: the muscle that opposes a given motion
- Stabilizers: provide stability by contracting to hold joints or segments of the body in place while others around it are free to move

Planes of Body Movement

Personal trainers should understand planes of body movement in order to diversify workouts and focus on all muscles, even smaller, weaker, or assistive muscles. While the body does not necessarily operate in an isolated plane of motion, exercises should focus on combining movements and planes of motion so that the client can more seamlessly flow from movement to movement with more flexibility and to prevent muscle imbalances. Understanding the proper form in which movement should occur in the planes also helps personal trainers notice improper movements and correct them. The planes of movement of the body include the following:

- Frontal/Coronal: splits the body into front and back sections
- Sagittal: splits the body into right and left sections
- Midsagittal: the specific instance of a sagittal plane that divides the body into equal right and left halves
- Transverse: splits the body into top and bottom sections

Interrelationships Among Center of Gravity, Base of Support, Balance, Stability, and Proper Spinal Alignment

The center of gravity is the location of a theoretical point that represents the total weight of an object. In most humans, the center of gravity is anterior to the second sacral vertebrae.

The base of support refers to the part of an object that serves as the supporting surface, often thought of as feet in contact with the ground. The base of support extends to mean the area between the feet as well, not just the physical structures of the body in contact with the supporting surface. Increasing the base of support makes it easier to be more stable and have an easier time balancing.

Balance is the ability to control the center of mass within the base of support without falling. The wider the base of support and the lower the center of gravity, the easier it is to maintain balance. This concept can be applied to squatting. Personal trainers can instruct clients to widen their base of support, squat back, and bring their hips back (as if they are sitting in a chair) in order to lower their center of mass without disturbing balance.

Stability is the ability to lean or deviate the body in one direction or another without changing base of support (taking a step or replanting the feet). Stability, like balance, is improved with a wider base of support. It can also be improved with core training.

Proper spinal alignment refers to the composition of the spine, which is composed of thirty-three (seven cervical, twelve thoracic, five lumbar, five sacral, and four coccygeal) vertebrae and the discs between them. There are normal curvatures of the spine in the sagittal plane: cervical and lumbar lordosis (convex anteriorly and concave posteriorly) and thoracic and sacral kyphosis (concave anteriorly and convex posteriorly). It is important to utilize good posture during resistance exercises to protect the spine from injury.

Irregular Curves of the Spine

Irregular curvatures of the spine can cause reduced range of motion, pain with high-impact exercise, and difficulty with certain movements. The personal trainer should be aware of the individual client's limitations and may need to rely more heavily on weight machines due to the greater support and reduced core stability needed with muscle isolation machines. There are three irregular curves of the spine:

- Lordosis: exaggerated curvature of the lumbar spine, which may cause discomfort, particularly during high-impact activities and standing for extended periods of time
- Scoliosis: lateral (often an "S") curvature of the spine
- Kyphosis: exaggerated curvature of the thoracic spine

Aerobic and Anaerobic Energy Systems

ATP is the energy molecule of the body and can be generated from the ATP-PC and glycolysis anaerobic (without oxygen) and aerobic (with oxygen) metabolic pathways.

- ATP-PC system: anaerobic, uses ATP stored in muscles, sufficient only for about ten-second high-intensity bouts of activity

- Glycolysis: anaerobic, creates ATP from carbohydrates (glucose) metabolism, used for two-three minutes of high intensity activity, but produces lactic acid as a byproduct

- Aerobic (Krebs cycle): aerobic, ATP generated through breakdown of carbohydrates, fats and, to a lesser degree, proteins, supplies energy during long duration endurance activities and used when the other energy systems are depleted or insufficient

Normal Acute Response to Cardiovascular and Resistance Training

At the onset of cardiovascular exercise, heart rate, blood pressure, and ventilation all increase immediately in healthy individuals in order to increase oxygen intake and transport, transitioning the body from anaerobic to aerobic energy systems. This same response is seen with resistance training,

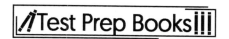

although these physiological variables do not typically remain elevated as the exercise session progresses because of the greater reliance on anaerobic metabolism for energy.

Normal Chronic Adaptations to Cardiovascular and Resistance Training

Heart and skeletal muscle hypertrophy is one of the chronic adaptations with regular cardiovascular and resistance training, respectively. With cardiovascular training, as the heart enlarges, the chamber sizes increase, allowing for a greater stroke volume and cardiac output. This also enables the heart to be more efficient, which lowers the resting heart rate and blood pressure as well as the submaximal exercise heart rate and blood pressure. It also increases exercise time and intensity tolerance. Total blood volume increases, reflecting both an increase in plasma volume and hemoglobin concentration. These circulatory adaptations increase the blood's oxygen-carrying capacity as well as the rate of removal of metabolic byproducts, such as carbon dioxide and lactate. The liver also becomes better able to metabolize the lactate from glycolysis, so that it can be used more effectively for energy. Endurance performance is often enhanced due to metabolic adaptations such as increased muscle glycogen storage and a greater reliance on fat (rather than carbohydrates) as an energy substrate at higher workloads. The ability to metabolize fat at greater intensities further spares glycogen, which can delay "hitting the wall"—a rapid onset of fatigue when the finite stores are consumed in the later stages of an endurance bout. Vasculature also increases, so blood perfusion of muscles improves. Other positive adaptations include increased bone mineral density, improvements in body composition, and neural adaptations.

Chronic resistance training also affords strength, power, and coordination improvements as well as greater efficiency of the anaerobic systems. Nervous system adaptations occur quickly with training as motor units (an alpha motor neuron from the spine and all of the skeletal muscle fibers it innervates) become conditioned to activate more quickly and more often, increasing the efficiency of stimulating muscle fibers to contract. As more motor units activate together and coordinate, a higher percentage of fibers in a muscle contract simultaneously, improving strength. In fact, many of the earliest strength improvements noticed in resistance training programs are due to these neural adaptations rather than muscle hypertrophy (which takes four to eight weeks to occur). A client can experience increased strength and power very quickly as a result of training. Over time, muscle fibers increase in size and bone mineral density increases in load-bearing bones, helping mitigate age-related bone and muscle loss.

Physiologic Response to Warm-Up and Cool-Down

Warm-ups and cool-downs are important components of the workout and help reduce injury risk by gradually transitioning the cardiovascular and musculoskeletal systems of the body between levels of rest and activity. They also improve joint range of motion by increasing the extensibility of connective tissue.

Effective warm-ups should begin by stoking the cardiovascular system with gentle, total body movements to start increasing heart rate and blood pressure, which better circulates oxygen, nutrients, and blood to the muscles. Specific muscles can be targeted (those that the training session will be focusing on) as the warm-up progresses.

The transition from exercise back to resting conditions is equally important and is the function of a cool-down. Without a proper cool-down to slow the heart rate gradually, cardiac dysrhythmias and feelings of dizziness can occur due to the decrease in venous return.

Soreness vs. Overtraining

Acute muscle fatigue occurs while the exercise is taking place and subsides when it stops. In contrast, delayed onset muscle soreness (DOMS) typically begins to develop twelve to twenty-four hours post-exercise, peaking twenty-four to seventy-two hours after the session, especially after high-repetition eccentric exercises like downhill running. DOMS likely develops as a result of microscopic damage to muscle fibers as a side effect of the repair process.

Overtraining is a condition that occurs when an individual trains with too much frequency and/or intensity, causing fatigue, greater injury risk, sleep issues, changes in appetite or body weight, lack of motivation, depression or moodiness, and performance decline. Signs of overtraining also include an elevated resting heart rate, soreness that does not resolve within a day or two after exercise (as is normal with resistance training), and an increased susceptibility to illness. The personal trainer should be aware of the client's volume, recovery, and intensity (both during sessions and on his/her own time) and use effective and continual communication, monitoring physiologic responses to workouts to prevent overtraining.

Effects of Rest, Submaximal Exercise, and Maximal Exercise

Adequate rest between bouts of high intensity activity, as well as between training sessions and whole training cycles, is an integral component of a program. Rest or recovery prevents overtraining, injuries, performance decline, and even weight gain. While eager clients may not understand the benefits of rest or may want to push their bodies too hard, the personal trainer should educate them on the need for rest to mitigate exercise's stress on bodily systems and prepare it for subsequent demands.

Routine submaximal exercise improves cardiovascular, musculoskeletal, respiratory, nervous, and metabolic systems of the body.

Maximal exercise carries a high risk of injury without significant benefit so it should be reserved primarily for testing/competition purposes. Main benefits beyond the upper thresholds of submaximal training are largely related to conditioning the mind to endure the physiological challenge imposed on the body.

Muscular Strength and Endurance

Lifting heavier weights for fewer repetitions (one to eight) induces muscular strength gains, while lifting lighter weights for more repetitions (eight or more) improves muscular endurance. Both are important for safe and successful performance of activities of daily living (ADLs). Lifting maximal weight carries a higher risk of injury and should be reserved for healthy patients at certain parts of a training cycle with adequate rest.

Blood Pressure Responses

It is important to be aware of blood pressure (BP) changes during exercise, especially with the increasing number of people with hypertension. The following are the blood pressure responses:

- Acute exercise: As exercise intensity increases, there is a linear increase in systolic BP, while diastolic may decrease slightly or remain unchanged due to the decreased peripheral resistance.

- Chronic exercise: Resting BP may decrease, and BP is lower at a given level of submaximal work.

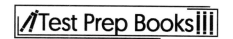

- Postural changes: Exercise may produce hypotensive response because of the reduced aortic pressure and improved pliability of blood vessels. If BP gets very low, clients may experience orthotic hypotension (dizziness when standing). Trainers should encourage fluid intake and have clients change positions more gradually.

Muscle Actions

Personal trainers need to be familiar with muscle actions and be cognizant that they should incorporate all types of contractions into workouts for optimal functional strength.

- Isotonic: a muscle contraction that exerts a constant tension
- Isometric: a muscle contraction in which there is no change in muscle length
- Isokinetic: a muscle contraction that moves through the range of motion at a constant speed
- Concentric: a muscle contraction with shortening, such as the biceps in the lifting portion of the biceps curl
- Eccentric: a lengthening muscle contraction, such as the biceps in the lowering the weight portion of the movement, frequently the cause of DOMS

Major Muscles

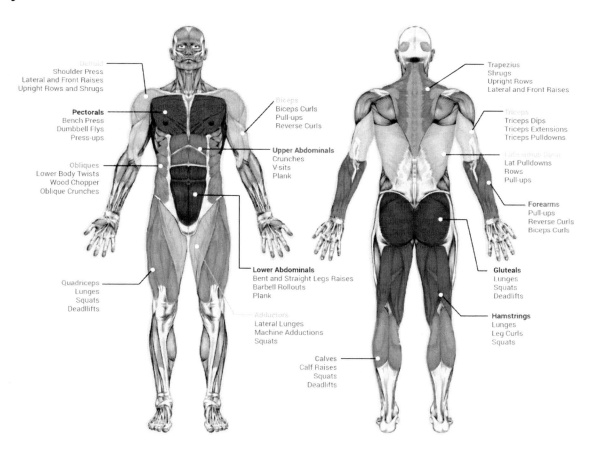

Trainers should not only be aware of muscle names, but also their origins, insertions, primary action, and nerve innervation. An understanding of these criteria can help in identifying injuries. It can also help ensure that exercises are targeting all muscles to maximize strength, strengthen stabilizing muscles, and provide proximal stability for functional distal mobility.

- Upper body muscles: trapezius, pectoralis major, deltoids, serratus anterior, latissimus dorsi, biceps, triceps, rectus abdominis, internal and external obliques, erector spinae, rhomboids, flexor carpi radialis

- Lower body muscles: iliopsoas, gluteus maximus, quadriceps, piriformis, hamstrings, adductors, abductors, soleus, gastrocnemius

Major Bones

Knowledge of bone anatomy enables the trainer to understand the bones involved in joint motions and the bones that may be implicated in certain orthopedic injuries, which is important when communicating with physicians. There are different types of bones. Flat bones, like the cranial bones of the skull and the sternum, protect internal organs. Long bones, like the femur and tibia, support weight and facilitate movement. Short bones, like the carpal bones in the wrist, provide stability and some movement. Irregular bones also protect structures like the vertebrae over the spinal cord. Lastly, sesamoid bones, like the patella, protect tendons from stress.

- Upper body bones: clavicle, scapula, sternum, humerus, carpals, ulna, radius, metacarpals, vertebrae, ribs

- Lower body bones: ilium, ischium, pubis, femur, fibula, tibia, metatarsals, tarsals

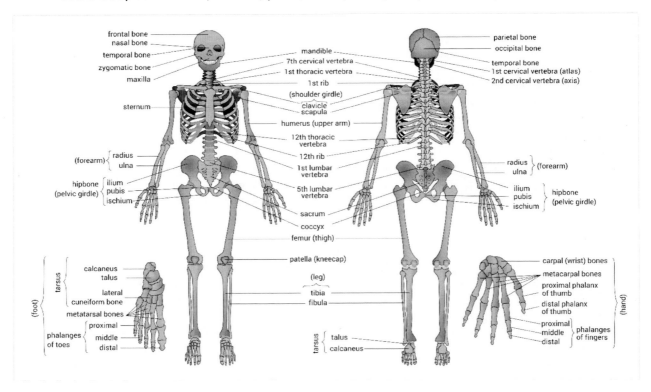

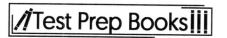

Joint Classifications

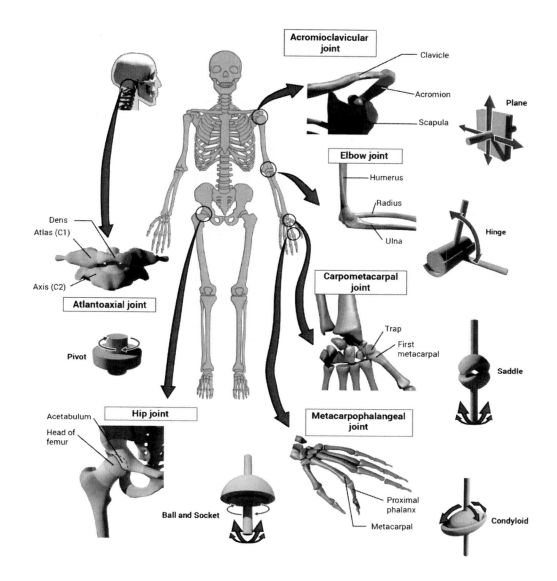

Joints can be classified based on structure of how the bones are connected:

- Fibrous joints: bones joined by fibrous tissue and that lack a joint cavity, e.g., sutures of the skull

- Cartilaginous joints: bones joined by cartilage and lack a joint cavity, e.g., the pubic symphysis

- Synovial joints: bones separated by a fluid-containing joint cavity with articular cartilage covering the ends of the bone and forming a capsule

- Plane joints: flat surfaces that allow gliding and transitional movements, e.g., intercarpal joints

- Hinge joints: cylindrical projection that nests in a trough-shaped structure, single plane of movement (e.g. the elbow)

- Pivot joints: rounded structure that sits into a ring-like shape, allowing uniaxial rotation of the bone around the long axis (e.g. radius head on ulna)

- Condyloid joints: oval articular surface that nests in a complementary depression, allowing all angular movements (e.g. the wrist)

- Saddle joints: articular surfaces that both have complementary concave and convex areas, allowing more movement than condyloid joints (e.g. the thumb)

- Ball-and-socket joints: spherical structure that fits in a cuplike structure, allowing multiaxial movements (e.g. the shoulder)

Primary Action and Joint Range of Motion

Each type of joint permits different movements, controlled by the shape of the joint and the muscles surrounding it. Personal trainers should be aware of these movements and the normal ROM to ensure that clients are performing exercises safely, are within a healthy range, and are utilizing a variety of motions to optimize health and muscular balance. Ball-and-socket joints, like the shoulder and hip, are the most mobile and allow flexion, extension, abduction, adduction, internal and external rotation, and circumduction. The elbow is a hinge joint and allows flexion and extension. Intervertebral joints are cartilaginous and allow flexion, extension, lateral flexion, and rotation. The ankle has a hinge joint (dorsiflexion, plantarflexion) and a gliding joint (inversion, eversion).

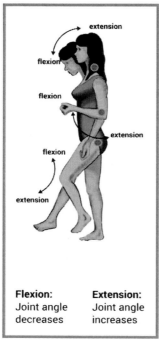

Flexion: Joint angle decreases

Extension: Joint angle increases

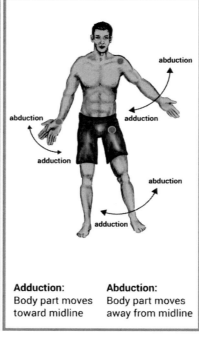

Adduction: Body part moves toward midline

Abduction: Body part moves away from midline

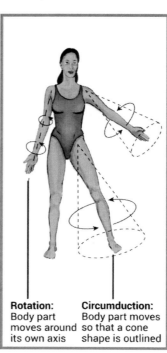

Rotation: Body part moves around its own axis

Circumduction: Body part moves so that a cone shape is outlined

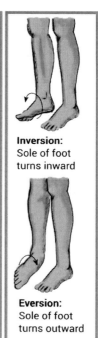

Inversion: Sole of foot turns inward

Eversion: Sole of foot turns outward

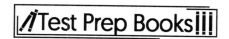

Muscle Terms

- Hypertrophy: increase in muscle fiber cross-sectional area, often an adaptation from strength training, an increase in fiber size, not fiber number, muscle strength gained from resistance training mostly due to hypertrophy

- Atrophy: reduction in muscle size due to a decrease in fiber cross-sectional area (opposite of hypertrophy) often due to physical inactivity, disease, nutritional inadequacies, or a disease of the muscle or nerve supplying the muscle

- Hyperplasia: an increase in muscle size due to an increase in the number of muscle fibers

Components of Physical Fitness

A well-rounded program addresses all five components of health-related physical fitness:

- Cardiovascular fitness: capacity of circulatory and respiratory systems to supply oxygen during continued activity
- Muscular strength: force capability of a muscle
- Muscular endurance: ability to maintain level of muscular work without fatigue
- Body composition: relative amounts of body fat, muscle, bone, and other tissues
- Flexibility: permitted joint range of motion

Normal Chronic Physiological Adaptations Associated with Cardiovascular, Resistance, and Flexibility Training

Cardiovascular training increases the number of mitochondria and oxidative enzymes on a cellular level, as well as facilitates an increase in capillaries and muscle blood flow, all leading to improved aerobic metabolism. Muscle glycogen storage increases, as well as the enhanced ability to metabolize fat for energy to spare glycogen stores. There are increases in cardiac output and stroke volume (due to increased plasma volume and left ventricle size) during exercise, as well as a lower resting and submaximal heart rate and blood pressure. VO_2 max and lactate threshold can increase as can the maximal pulmonary ventilation rate.

Resistance training increases skeletal muscle force due to hypertrophy (increase in cross-sectional area of muscle fibers) and greater, more coordinated fiber recruitment due to neural adaptations. There is also increased strength and size of tendons and ligaments, ATP-PC and glycogen stores, and improvements in lactate utilization.

Flexibility training increases the elasticity and resting length of muscle and connective tissues and joint ROM before the stretch reflex is initiated (muscle spindle adaptation), reducing injury risk.

Exercise Testing Precautions

In certain circumstances, testing is not safe, and there are absolute contraindications. It is important for the personal trainer to heed the advice of medical professionals and work with physicians specifically trained in exercise testing in those cases where physician supervision of assessments is recommended. It is prudent to err on the side of caution, such as choosing submaximal tests over maximal tests.

Absolute contraindications	Relative contraindications*
Post myocardial infarction (two days)	Electrolyte abnormalities
Inability to obtain consent	Atrial fibrillation or high-degree AV block
Physical impairment that would preclude safe testing	Coronary stenosis, valvular heart disease
Acute illness (myocarditis, endocarditis, infection, pulmonary embolism, renal failure) that could be aggravated by exercise	Tachycardia or Bradyarrhythmia, hypertrophic cardiomyopathy
Uncontrolled cardiac arrhythmias, aortic stenosis, symptomatic heart failure	Inability to cooperate or mental impairment affecting comprehension/informed consent
Unstable angina	

* If benefits are deemed to outweigh risks, relative contraindications can be superseded.

Test Termination	
Absolute indications	**Relative indications**
Drop in systolic BP below baseline despite workload increase	Increasing chest discomfort
New or increasing chest pain	Fatigue, breathlessness, wheezing, cramping
Client's request to stop	Minor heart arrhythmias
Serious arrhythmias	EKG changes such as QRS axis shift
Technical difficulties with EKG or BP monitoring	Bundle branch block
CNS symptoms: dizziness, ataxia, etc.	Perceived maximal effort or achievement of clinical end points
Signs of poor peripheral perfusion, cyanosis	

After sudden test termination, place patient supine or seated and continue to monitor blood pressure and EKG for six to eight minutes. If test ends comfortably and normally, the patient should walk or slowly and gradually cool down to bring physiologic parameters back to resting value.

Body Composition Techniques

Body composition assessments are an important parameter to track and measure, particularly because some clients may lose body fat, but make gains in lean body mass through training. Thus, they see little progress on the scale, despite larger improvements in health. There are varieties of techniques for assessing body fat, each inherent with its own set of pros and cons:

Skinfold measurements: caliper measurements of subcutaneous fat from pinches of skin at specific body sites, plugged into equations to estimate body fat percentage

Pros: easy to conduct in the field, more accurate than BMI, inexpensive

Cons: uncomfortable for clients emotionally (given some immodest access sites) and somewhat physically, requires trainer skilled in obtaining accurate measurements

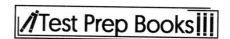

Plethysmography (BOD POD®): special laboratory tool, uses air displacement to calculate volume of the body along with weight to determine body fat

Pros: highly accurate, as much so as hydrostatic weighing, but easier to administer and fast

Cons: not highly available, more expensive than field tests, can be impractical for regular reassessments

Bioelectrical impedance: uses the principle that fat mass and fat free mass have different resistances to electrical current, which can be measured to report body fat percentage

Pros: very inexpensive devices, non-invasive, comfortable for clients, fairly accurate

Cons: sensitive to body hydration status, requiring restrictions on client's eating/drinking (shouldn't eat or drink for at least thirty minutes), exercising (none for at least twelve hours), drinking alcohol (none for at least 48 hours), and caffeine intake (abstain prior to test)

Infrared: fat mass and fat-free mass assessed via a specialized infrared-light-emitting probe placed against an area of the body

Pros: non-invasive, top-of-the-line laboratory devices, very accurate

Cons: may overestimate body fat in lean people and underestimate in overweight, commercially available devices not as accurate

Dual-energy X-ray absorptiometry (DEXA): measures bone mineral density fat mass via a specialized infrared-light-emitting probe placed against an area of the body.

Pros: most accurate and easy to administer, done in clothes, quick results, also assesses bone mineral density, measures entire body, not just estimating based on certain sites

Cons: requires trip to physician/laboratory, can be expensive, not recommended for pregnant women due to x-ray

Circumference measurements: measurements with measuring tape at specific body sites, plugged into equations to estimate body fat percentage

Pros: can be more accurate than skinfolds on very obese clients, easy to administer in the field, less skill involved than skinfold measurements so often less measurement error, inexpensive

Cons: typically not as accurate of an estimate as skinfold or laboratory tests

Fitness Testing Protocols

There are a variety of field-based and laboratory tests available for each of the five components of fitness. Selecting the appropriate method involves weighing the inherent pros and cons for each test modality and taking into account each client's characteristics such as age, health status, fitness level, availability, goals, physical impairments, and skill level.

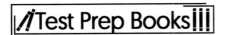

Common Assessments

Cardiovascular fitness: YMCA step test, Rockport Walk Test, Astrand-Rhyming or YMCA Cycle Test, 1-mile run

- Muscular strength: bench press or leg press 1 repetition max (RM), 3RM
- Muscular endurance: push-up test, one-minute sit-up test
- Body composition: skinfold, BOD-POD, DEXA, circumferences
- Flexibility: sit-and-reach test

Interpretation of Fitness Test Results

Each of the recommended fitness assessments has standards upon which the personal trainer can compare a client's results. Norm-referenced standards, such as VO_2 max score, compare the client's performance against that of other similar people, and scores are presented in percentiles. The fiftieth percentile indicates the client performed better than half of the comparative population and worse than half. It is important that the trainer reports not just the percentile score, but educates the client on his or her score's relative value.

Criterion-referenced standards are based on research and normative-based achievement levels of health and fitness that, if reached, would predict lower disease risk for the client. Universal agreement of the specific, minimal health standards and cutoffs does not exist, but many tests have enough consensus to set goal levels for a client. For deconditioned clients, the personal trainer should try to focus them on improving their scores from baseline, regardless as to how far from "average" or "healthy" they are, to avoid feelings of discouragement and lowering self-esteem.

Recommended Order of Fitness Assessments

After the client has completed the health questionnaire, provided informed consent, completed the initial interview to discuss goals, fitness level, and any injuries, and has received any necessary medical clearance, testing can begin. There is not a mandated sequence of assessments that the personal trainer must follow, and often, the exact order is determined by the setting and available equipment. If possible, it is often best to do resting measures prior to exertional ones to avoid assessments being negatively affected by fatigue. In order to prevent injury, flexibility should be done at the end after muscles have had adequate warm-up time.

- Resting measurements (heart rate, blood pressure, and weight to get a resting baseline)
- Body Composition (circumference measurements, skinfolds, BMI)
- Cardiovascular Fitness (Step Test or one mile run)
- Muscular strength and endurance assessments (Push-ups)
- Flexibility (Sit and Reach Test or V-Sit Test)

Documentation of Abnormal Symptoms and Subsequent Physician Referral

Personal trainers are allied health professionals, and to avoid operating outside their scope of practice, they should refer clients to physicians and other healthcare clinicians when clients display or mention certain signs and symptoms of orthopedic, cardiorespiratory, metabolic, and neurologic issues. When in doubt, it is prudent for the trainer to seek the advice of healthcare professionals. Any and all documentation of symptoms (e.g., knee pain with squatting, dizziness with exertion) and objective

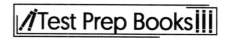

measurements (e.g., heart rate or blood pressure before, during, or after exercise) should be sent with the referral along with a clear, concise narrative detailing the concern.

Referral to a Physician

Trainers should be prepared to refer clients to local physicians for a variety of issues clients may experience, ranging from medical clearance to musculoskeletal issues. HIPAA policies and confidentiality should be exercised while communicating the pertinent health information. After the referral has been established, the trainer and physician should have ongoing communication about the client's ability to participate in the exercise program as well as to provide updates and any necessary modifications.

Assessing Intensity During Exercise

Personal trainers can assess peripheral pulses, typically at either the carotid or radial arteries, and teach clients how to palpate these areas for a pulse correctly. The common carotid artery is located on the side of the neck in the groove between the trachea and hyoid muscles. The pulse can be palpated just under the anterior edge of the sternocleidomastoid. The radial pulse is taken on the thumb side (lateral side) of the wrist.

After the pulse location is correctly identified, the index and middle fingers are placed over the site, counting pulsations for a given time interval (ten, fifteen, thirty seconds) and extrapolating this number out for a one minute interval. Pulse counts are more accurate for longer intervals, but also slow down more noticeably the longer the interval since ceasing activity. The more intense the activity, the shorter the counting interval should be for greater accuracy. While less common in a fitness setting, heart rate can be measured at the brachial, femoral, popliteal, tibialis posterior, and dorsalis pedis arteries.

Rate of perceived exertion (RPE) can be used during exercise and testing as a subjective indicator of effort level, especially with older adults, those on HR-altering medications, and those in whom measuring heart rate is difficult. A six to twenty ("no exertion at all" to "maximum exertion") Borg scale is most commonly employed, with studies indicating that the threshold for improvements in cardiorespiratory fitness are at an RPE between twelve and sixteen ("hard" range).

Selecting Cardiovascular Assessments

There are a variety of cardiovascular assessments trainers can choose from, depending on client age, fitness level, health, interests, and testing environment. Field tests typically require minimal equipment and occur outside (i.e., "in the field"), such as the Rockport walk test, 1-mile run, or Step Test. Laboratory tests, such as the YMCA Cycle Ergometer test, require equipment. Health, fitness level, and injuries also factor into assessment selection. It may be safer and more successful for a sedentary client to do a submaximal test like the YMCA Cycle Ergometer test rather than a VO$_2$ max treadmill protocol, and a client with a sore knee would be better suited for a cycle rather than running test as well. Normal acute responses to cardiovascular exercise include increases in heart rate, blood pressure, stroke volume, respiration, and body temperature.

Circumference Measurements

Circumference measurements should be taken with a flexible plastic tape that is taut, but does not indent the skin. The personal trainer should measure all sites, record the values, and measure each specific area in order once, and then in the same order again.

Waist circumference (smallest circumference between xiphoid and umbilicus) alone has health-related criterion standards as abdominal obesity carries a greater risk for high blood pressure, metabolic syndrome, type 2 diabetes, high cholesterol, CAD, and premature death. The standards for high risk are ≥ 102 cm for men and ≥ 88 cm for women. The standards for low risk are < 80 cm for men and < 70 cm for women).

Waist-to-hip ratio is another commonly used marker of health. Other circumference sites are often taken to monitor over time with exercise training and to assess how body shape changes. Such sites include the upper arm, buttocks, calf, forearm, abdomen, and mid-thigh. The personal trainer should be consistent with measurement sites to avoid contributing to error.

Skinfold Measurement Sites

Skinfold measurements should be taken precisely, on dry skin, and with an experienced tester. Two measurements should be taken per site, both on the right side of the body, with values no more than 2 mm or 10 percent difference. The following sites are typically used:

- Chest: diagonal fold halfway for men and one-third for women of the distance from anterior axillary line and nipple

- Midaxilla: vertical fold on midaxillary line at xiphoid level

- Triceps: vertical fold on midline of triceps, halfway between acromion and olecranon with elbow extended and relaxed

- Subscapula: diagonal fold on line connecting inferior angle of scapula to a point 0.8 inches from the medial border

- Abdomen: vertical fold one-inch lateral to umbilicus

- Suprailium: vertical fold above iliac crest in line with anterior axillary line

- Thigh: anterior vertical fold halfway between hip and knee joints

Selecting Safe Muscular Assessments

Trainers should carefully review medical history and all of the prescreening stratification for any contraindications to testing and review any necessary safety precautions, such as physician supervision, during testing. The benefits of selected tests must always outweigh potential risks. Client factors—including health status, such as any current illness or injuries, functional capacity, age, sex, and pre-training status—should be considered when selecting an appropriate assessment. For example, a bench press 1RM test may not be appropriate for an older adult with shoulder pain. In such a case, a test at submaximal workloads to predict maximum would be a safer choice. It is normal for heart rate and blood pressure to increase during resistance exercise as the heart works to oxygenate and fuel the working muscles.

Selecting Safe Flexibility Assessments

To avoid injury, the muscles, ligaments, and tendons should be fully warmed-up prior to flexibility assessments. Pushing joints beyond the comfortable and normal range of motion can also cause injury,

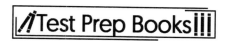

so clients should be instructed on how to complete the assessments and stretches, prior to attempting them. Flexibility will tend to improve with conditioning and consistency, although temperature, genetics, sex, and age determine certain limits of flexibility. Ballistic stretching should be avoided as it can injure muscles and tendons. With the sit-and-reach assessment, a moderate stretch may be felt in the low back, hamstrings, arms, and calves, but it should not feel painful.

Recognizing Postural Abnormalities

Trainers can screen for postural abnormalities such as kyphosis, lordosis, and scoliosis using a posture chart (a grid that the client stands in front of) or a plumb line. Scoliosis is a lateral curvature of the spine. A client with scoliosis will display unequal heights of posterior landmarks such as shoulder height or iliac crests. The posture grid helps provide an objective background for this assessment. Lordosis and kyphosis are exaggerated curves in the lumbar and cervical spine respectively and are best viewed from the side. A curvature of twenty to forty-five degrees is normal; beyond forty-five degrees is abnormal. Lumbar lordosis greater than sixty degrees is considered abnormal.

Delivering Assessment Results

The personal trainer must develop skill in communicating assessment results in a positive and professional manner. Clients are often anxious and vulnerable in early stages of starting the behavioral change of incorporating exercise, so it is critical to deliver results in a respectful, competent, and non-judgmental way. Trainers should maintain confidentiality and instill an environment of trust and empathy so that clients do not lose motivation and self-confidence or feel embarrassed.

Developing a Comprehensive Plan

After consideration of risk stratification, goals, test results, client availability, and commitment level, trainers should employ the FITT-VP framework to develop a plan for each component of fitness:

- Frequency: how often
- Intensity: effort (% of VO_2 max, % 1RM)
- Time: duration of exercise
- Type: mode (running, yoga, lifting weights)
- Volume: total amount
- Progress: advancement

Development of Fitness Plans

Developing the fitness plan is a comprehensive process that takes place after the client interview and risk stratification physical fitness assessments, as well as after discussions of goals, lifestyle, behavioral factors, and perceived barriers. Plans may include sessions that clients complete independently (i.e., in addition to scheduled training sessions with the trainer, depending on client goals, training experience, motivation, schedule, and budget). Plans should focus on S.M.A.R.T. goals, targeting all five areas of health-related fitness, with an emphasis on areas of greatest deficit and/or interest. Trainers should include a variety of exercise modalities to prevent boredom and to maximize functional fitness and include regularly scheduled reassessments. It should be noted that plans serve as a guideline and may need to be modified to accommodate injuries, illnesses, and unpredicted rates of improvement.

Health Behavior Modification Strategies to Meet Goals

Goal-setting should include both short and long term goals and begin with some simply-achievable goals to develop a feeling of mastery and success and build self-confidence. Through positive reinforcement and abstaining from punishment, trainers can influence a client's behavior and exercise adherence. Motivation affects behavior as well. Intrinsically motivated clients, or those with self-determination, enjoy the process of the exercise itself and therefore may maintain their health behaviors more easily than externally motivated clients, who exercise for the sake of achieving some sort of reward. Self-efficacy, or the client's confidence in his or her ability to make the behavioral change, also influences goal achievement and can be improved with modeling, performance accomplishments, and verbal encouragement.

Reassessment

Goals and progress can be measured at regular intervals to be compared to a baseline, typically every four to twelve weeks, depending on the frequency of sessions, goal difficulty, and client personality. Trainers should track workouts and record detailed information about sessions, including weights, reps, rest intervals, RPE, modifications made to workouts or exercises based on pain, and fatigue. Trainers should be mindful of reassessing each component of fitness (cardiovascular, muscular strength/endurance, flexibility, and body composition), noting which areas are in need of renewed focus.

Practice Questions

1. Which of the following is NOT considered one of the five main components of health-related physical fitness?
    a. Muscular power
    b. Flexibility
    c. Muscular endurance
    d. Body composition

2. Which of the following statements are true about medical clearance prior to participating in an exercise-training program?
    a. All clients need medical clearance from a physician prior to participation in an exercise-training program.
    b. Only clients with diagnosed cardiovascular, respiratory, or metabolic diseases need clearance prior to participation.
    c. Children, adolescents, men less than forty-five years, and women less than fifty-five years who do not have CAD risk factors/symptoms or known disease and who did not answer "yes" to any questions on the PAR-Q do not need clearance.
    d. Children, adolescents, men less than fifty years, and women less than fifty-five years who do not have CAD risk factors/symptoms or a known disease and who did not answer "yes" to any questions on the PAR-Q do not need clearance.

3. The Client-Trainer agreement form should include all of the following EXCEPT:
    a. Cost-structure for sessions
    b. Cancellation policy
    c. Expectations of both parties
    d. Risk stratification information

4. What is the criteria of obesity that counts as a positive risk factor for CAD?
    a. Waist circumference of > 100 cm
    b. BMI ≤ 29 kg/m^2
    c. Waist circumference of < 100 cm
    d. BMI ≥ 29 kg/m^2

5. Which of the following is a positive risk factor for CAD?
    a. Blood pressure reading of 130/90 mmHg
    b. Fasting blood glucose of ≥ 90 mg/dL confirmed by at least two separate measurements
    c. Current use of lipid-lowering medications
    d. Death of father at age sixty-six from myocardial infarction

6. Which of the following is the best definition for intermittent claudication?
    a. Tissue swelling as a result of an imbalance between fluid coming out of circulation in blood vessels into tissues or back into circulation from tissue
    b. Dizziness upon standing that resolves with sitting or lying down
    c. Microscopic tissue damage from eccentric exercise that usually appears twenty-four hours after exercise
    d. An achy, cramping feeling typically of the lower legs that may come and go with exercise due to occlusion of blood vessels

7. Which of the following lists of joint types is in the correct order for increasing amounts of permitted motion (least mobile to most mobile)?
a. Hinge, condyloid, saddle
b. Saddle, hinge, condyloid
c. Saddle, condyloid, hinge
d. Hinge, saddle, condyloid

8. In order to be stratified as low risk, a client must meet which of the following conditions?
I. Male less than forty-five years of age or female less than fifty-five years
II. Asymptomatic
III. Have no risk factors for cardiovascular or pulmonary disease
IV. Have one risk factor for cardiovascular or pulmonary disease

a. I and III only
b. II and III only
c. I, II, and III
d. I, II, and IV

9. Which type of diabetes results from little to no insulin production?
a. Type I
b. Type II
c. Both Type I and Type II
d. Neither Type I nor Type II

10. Which of the following is the correct order of behavioral change stages according to the trans-theoretical model?
a. Pre-contemplation, Contemplation, Preparation, Action, Maintenance
b. Preparation, Pre-contemplation, Contemplation, Maintenance, Action
c. Preparation, Contemplation, Pre-contemplation, Action, Maintenance
d. Pre-contemplation, Preparation, Contemplation, Action, Maintenance

11. Which is the most likely stage in the trans-theoretical model for a client to say, "I exercised once last week, and I'll try to exercise twice this week"?
a. Preparation
b. Pre-contemplation
c. Contemplation
d. Action

12. Which of the following neurotransmitters helps strengthen the synaptic pathways involved in learning a behavior through reinforcement?
a. Epinephrine
b. Serotonin
c. Norepinephrine
d. Dopamine

13. Match the behavioral change model with the best descriptive choice.
    a. Social Cognitive Theory: addresses relationships; behaviors, such as a client's motivation to exercise, are shaped by interpersonal relations, the surrounding environment, community, policy, and law.
    b. Health Belief Model: the perceived seriousness of a potential health problem is the main predictors of behavioral change.
    c. Socio-Ecological Model: clients actively shape their lives and learn by thinking, feeling, reflecting, and observing themselves in a social context.
    d. Theory of Planned Behavior: the client's level of motivation for behavioral change is shaped by his or her attitudes and behaviors that will most like occur in the allotted timeframe

14. Ligaments connect what?
    a. Muscle to muscle
    b. Bone to bone
    c. Bone to muscle
    d. Muscle to tendon

15. Which of the following reflects the correct blood flow pathway (heart-valve-vessel)?
    a. Right atrium, left atrium, right ventricle, mitral valve, left ventricle, aorta
    b. Right atrium, mitral valve, right ventricle, systemic circulation, left atrium, left ventricle, aorta
    c. Right atrium, right ventricle, left atrium, tricuspid valve, left ventricle, aorta
    d. Right atrium, right ventricle, pulmonary circulation, left atrium, mitral valve, left ventricle, aorta

16. Which of the following terms means "movement away from the body's midline"?
    a. Abduction
    b. Adduction
    c. Pronation
    d. Supination

17. What muscle is the primary antagonist in knee flexion?
    a. Hamstrings
    b. Quadriceps
    c. Gastrocnemius
    d. Tibialis anterior

18. In what plane does shoulder flexion occur?
    a. Sagittal
    b. Frontal
    c. Transverse
    d. Coronal

19. In what region of the spine is the lordosis often exaggerated as an irregular spinal curve?
    a. Cervical
    b. Thoracic
    c. Lumbar
    d. Sacral

20. What is the primary energy pathway for ATP production for an intense two-minute bout of activity?
    a. Aerobic metabolism
    b. Krebs cycle
    c. Glycolysis
    d. ATP-PC system

21. Which of the following is NOT an adaptation to chronic cardiovascular exercise?
    a. Increased heart chambers' sizes
    b. Increased stroke volume
    c. Increased cardiac output
    d. Increased submaximal heart rate

22. Which of the following is true about delayed onset muscle soreness (DOMS)?
    a. It typically peaks twenty-four to seventy-two hours post-workout, especially after eccentric exercises.
    b. It typically peaks twenty-four to seventy-two hours post-workout, especially after concentric exercises.
    c. It typically peaks twelve to twenty-four hours post-workout, especially after eccentric exercises.
    d. It typically peaks twelve to twenty-four hours post-workout, especially after concentric exercises.

23. Pectoralis major is doing what type of contraction during a pushup?
    a. Isokinetic
    b. Isometric
    c. Isotonic
    d. Eccentric

24. Which of the following types of joints are correctly matched with the anatomic joint example given?
    I. Cartilaginous: pubic symphysis
    II. Saddle: thumb carpal-metacarpal
    III. Plane: sutures in skull
    IV. Pivot: radial head on ulna

    a. Choices I, II, III
    b. Choices I, II, IV
    c. Choices I, III, IV
    d. All are correct

25. Which of the following is NOT an absolute indication to terminate an exercise test?
    a. New chest pain
    b. Cyanosis
    c. Client's request to stop
    d. Increasing chest discomfort

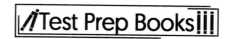

26. Tom is a new client. He is forty-two years old, a non-smoker, and enjoys golfing. He is healthy except for mild lateral epicondylitis and takes a beta-blocker. He has done his initial interview, clearance, and assessments. Which of the following guidelines would you give him for target effort range for his cardiovascular workouts for gains in aerobic fitness?
   a. Aim for twelve to fifteen RPE
   b. Aim for fifteen to eighteen RPE
   c. Aim for a heart rate of 106-142 bpm
   d. Aim for a heart rate of 150-180 bpm

27. In which order would a strength coach recommend administering the following assessments?
   a. Skinfold, push-up test, step test, 1RM bench press, sit-and-reach
   b. Skinfold, step test, push-up test, 1RM bench press, sit-and-reach
   c. Skinfold, sit-and-reach, step test, 1RM bench press, push-up test
   d. Skinfold, 1RM bench press, push-up test, step test, sit-and-reach

28. How often is reassessment of fitness testing recommended?
   a. Every two to three weeks
   b. Annually
   c. Every three to four months
   d. Every four to twelve weeks

29. Tim is a twenty-one-year-old college student who plays on the baseball team. He is coming to you for strengthening. He is 70 inches tall and weighs 160 pounds. He doesn't smoke, and both parents are healthy. He was diagnosed with Type 1 Diabetes at age eight, but his blood glucose is normal with insulin injections. His blood pressure is 105/68 mmHg, and his total cholesterol is 170 mg/dL. He reports no symptoms and can train after practice and on weekends.
In what risk category is Tim?
   a. No risk
   b. Low risk
   c. Moderate risk
   d. High risk

30. Sarah is a twenty-three-year-old client, who lives with both parents. She is 64 inches tall and weighs 128 pounds. Her blood pressure today is 116/75 mmHg, and her total cholesterol is 170 mg/dL. LDL is 120, and blood glucose is 82 mg/dL. She dances or plays volleyball most days of the week and smokes, but only on the weekends with friends.
How many risk factors for CAD does Sarah have?
   a. Zero
   b. One
   c. Two
   d. Three

31. A client's confidence in his or her ability to make the behavioral change is known as what?
   a. Self-determination
   b. Self-esteem
   c. Self-efficacy
   d. Determination

32. Tina is a fifty-eight-year-old sedentary female coming to you to "get in shape" since she "hasn't worked out since college." She is 180 pounds and 5'4," with a BMI of 30.9. She has no personal history of heart disease and quit smoking three years ago, but her mother had a myocardial infarction at the age of sixty-six. Tina's blood pressure is consistently 135/85 mm Hg, total cholesterol is 180 mg/dL with an HDL level of 30 mg/dL, and fasting blood glucose is 90 mg/dL.
How many risk factors for CAD does Tina have?
   a. Two
   b. Three
   c. Four
   d. Five

33. Which of the following skinfolds sites should be taken with a diagonal pinch/fold?
   a. Thigh
   b. Sub-scapula
   c. Triceps
   d. Abdomen

34. Which of the following is possibly a marker seen in someone with a risk of metabolic disease?
   a. Female waist circumference > 85 cm
   b. Triglyceride levels of 160 mg/dL
   c. HDL cholesterol of 50 mg/dL
   d. Fasting glucose levels of 105 mg/dL

35. Balance is facilitated by _____ the base of support and _____ the center of mass.
   a. Widening, lowering
   b. Widening, raising
   c. Lowering, widening
   d. Raising, raising

36. Which of the following may indicate trainer-client incompatibility?
   a. The client has never exercised before, and the trainer is a competitive athlete.
   b. The client is male, and the trainer is female.
   c. The client prefers to text and email, but the trainer likes talking on the phone or in person.
   d. The client is available to train weekdays, but the trainer only has weekend availability.

37. The FITT-VP framework for developing a comprehensive fitness plan stands for which of the following?
   a. Flexibility, Intensity, Time, Type, Variety, Purpose
   b. Fervency, Integrity, Time, Type, Volume, Purpose
   c. Follow-up, Intensity, Time, Type, Validity, Progress
   d. Frequency, Intensity, Time, Type, Volume, Progression

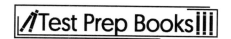

38. Paul is a thirty-eight-year-old recreational runner training for a local 10k. He is running five days a week and feeling good, but he wants to train with you to prevent injury. He is 72 inches tall and weighs 225 pounds. He takes Lipitor and a multivitamin. His blood pressure is 112/70 mmHg. His total cholesterol is 210 mg/dL. His father and mother are both alive, but his uncle died at age fifty from a stroke. Paul does not smoke or drink. He has medical clearance from his physical last week to begin a strength-training program with you. Which of the following do you recommend for his cardiovascular assessment?

    a. Astrand-Rhyming cycle ergometer test
    b. 1.5 mile run test with physician present
    c. Rockport walk test
    d. Astrand-Rhyming cycle ergometer with physician present

Answer Key and Explanations

1. A: The five main components of health-related physical fitness are cardiovascular fitness, muscular strength/endurance, flexibility, body composition, and flexibility. Muscular power is related to exercise performance and is a measure of strength to speed. It isn't one of the five components of fitness that directly relates to health.

2. C: Clients who are apparently healthy are not required to get medical clearance prior to starting an exercise program. These include children, adolescents, men less than forty-five years, and women less than fifty-five years who do not have CAD risk factors or symptoms, any known disease, and who did not answer "yes" to any questions on the PAR-Q. Choices A and B are not correct, and D provides too high of an age cutoff for "apparently healthy males."

3. D: Risk stratification is not included on the trainer-client agreement. In fact, the agreement may be discussed and signed prior to stratifying the client. The personal trainer and client are under contract law, so the trainer-client agreement is a written document signed by both parties describing the services, the involved parties, and the expectations of each, as well as a timeline of delivery, cost, and payment including aspects such as the cancellation policy and contract termination.

4. A: Waist circumference greater than 100 cm or a BMI $\geq$ 30 kg/m^2 indicates obesity and meets the criteria as a positive risk factor of CAD. Although either alone counts as a positive risk factor, the trainer should bear in mind that the waist circumference is probably a greater warning sign since it is more directly assessing abdominal obesity (shown to be detrimental to health), while BMI can be elevated in muscular individuals and is looking at total body density, not abdominal size.

5. C: Current use of lipid-lowering medications is a positive sign of CAD, even if cholesterol levels are normalized with medication usage. Other positive signs include the following:

- Family history of myocardial infarction
- Coronary revascularization
- Sudden death in a first-degree relative before age fifty-five in males or sixty-five in females
- Cigarette smoking, current or past six months
- Taking anti-hypertensive medications or systolic blood pressure $\geq$ 140 mmHg or diastolic pressure $\geq$ 90 mmHg confirmed by at least two separate measurements on different occasions
- Total cholesterol > 200 mg/dL, LDL > 130 mg/dL or low HDL < 40 mg/dL
- Fasting blood glucose: $\geq$ 100 mg/dL confirmed by at least two separate measurements on different occasions
- Waist circumference of > 100cm (39 inches) or BMI $\geq$ 30 kg/m^2
- A sedentary lifestyle

6. D: Intermittent claudication is an achy, cramping feeling typically of the lower legs that may come and go with exercise due to occlusion of blood vessels. Edema is tissue swelling due to an imbalance between fluids coming out of circulation in blood vessels into tissues or back into circulation from tissue. Dizziness upon standing is orthostatic hypotension and may cause syncope. Delayed onset muscle soreness (DOMS) is microscopic tissue damage that appears twenty-four hours after exercise.

7. A: All three joint types given are synovial joints, allowing for a fair amount of movement (compared with fibrous and cartilaginous joints). Of the three given, hinge joints, such as the elbow, permit the

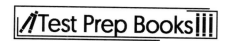

least motion because they are uniaxial and permit movement in only one plane. Saddle joints and condyloid joints both have reciprocating surfaces that mate with one another and allow a variety of motions in numerous planes, but saddle joints, such as the thumb carpal-metacarpal joint, allow more motion than condyloid joints. In saddle joints, two concave surfaces articulate, and in a condyloid joint, such as the wrist, a concave surface articulates with a convex surface, allowing motion in mainly two planes.

8. D: I, II, and IV. A client is low risk if he/she has one or fewer risk factors. The client should still be asymptomatic, less than the age of forty-five or fifty-five for men and women, respectively. Option III is no risk factors, but the client can have up to one. Thus, all of the other choices are incorrect.

9. A: Type I Diabetes results from little to no insulin production from the beta cells in the pancreas. It is an autoimmune disease and typically diagnosed in childhood. Type II Diabetes is not a result of inadequate production of insulin; typically, there is a sufficient amount in circulation, but the cells are not responsive to it.

10. A: The trans-theoretical model describes the client's process of getting ready to start exercise and consists of five stages: pre-contemplation, contemplation, preparation, action, and maintenance. In pre-contemplation, the client is not intending to take action toward changing physical activity and is not considering becoming physically active. During contemplation, the client intends to increase physical activity within the next six months. By the preparation stage, the client has developed a plan of action toward behavior change and will be making changes in the immediate future (next thirty days) and/or is inconsistently engaging in some amount of physical activity, but not at least thirty minutes of moderate-intensity activity for five or more days per week. In the action stage, the client is engaging in at least thirty minutes of moderate-intensity activity for five or more days per week but has done so for less than six months. Lastly, in maintenance, the client has been actively maintaining the changes made during the action stage; the new behaviors have been established for six months or more, and the client is now working to prevent relapse.

11. A: The preparation stage is the correct response because the client is inconsistently engaging in some amount of physical activity (in this case, once or twice per week) and not at least the recommended thirty minutes of moderate-intensity activity for five or more days per week. Note that in the contemplation stage, the client likely has not begun any sort of activity, not even once or twice a week, but is making plans to do so in the coming six months. In the action stage, the client would be regularly engaging in the activity and therefore would be doing it more often than the "once or twice a week" client in the example.

12. D: Dopamine helps strengthens the synaptic pathways involved in learning a behavior through reinforcement of the behavior. Several diseases are caused by disturbances of dopamine or its pathways. Parkinson's disease can result from too little dopamine activity, while Schizophrenia may be due to an excess of dopamine. Serotonin is the only other one of the choices that is a neurotransmitter, and involved in happiness/mood. Epinephrine and norepinephrine are hormones involved in the fight or flight response with stress.

13. B: The Health Belief Model is one in which the perceived seriousness of a potential health problem is the main predictor of behavioral change. The other models are not correctly matched with their meanings or are inaccurate. With the Theory of Planned Behavior, the client's level of motivation for behavioral change is shaped by his or her attitudes, subjective norms, and perceived control; behaviors in a timeframe are not part of this model. Social Cognitive Theory posits that clients actively shape their lives and learn by thinking, feeling, reflecting, and observing themselves in a social context. In the Socio-Ecological Model, behaviors, such as a client's motivation to exercise, are shaped by interpersonal relations, the surrounding environment, community, policy, and law.

14. B: Ligaments connect bone to bone. Tendons connect muscle to bone. Both are made of dense, fibrous connective tissue (primary Type 1 collagen) to give strength. However, tendons are more organized, especially in the long axis direction like muscle fibers themselves, and they have more collagen. This arrangement makes more sense because muscles have specific orientations of their fibers, so they contract in somewhat predictable directions. Ligaments are less organized and more of a woven pattern because bone connections are not as organized as bundles or muscle fibers, so ligaments must have strength in multiple directions to protect against injury.

15. D: Blood returning to the heart from the body enters the right atrium and then moves through the tricuspid valve into the right ventricle. After filling, the right ventricle contracts, and the tricuspid valve closes, pushing blood through the pulmonary semilunar valve into the pulmonary arteries for pulmonary circulation, after which it enters the left atrium. Contraction of the left atrium moves blood through the bicuspid valve into the left ventricle (the largest heart chamber). When the bicuspid valve closes and the left ventricle contracts, blood is forced into the aortic valve through the aorta and on to systemic circulation.

16. A: Abduction is movement away from the body's midline (out to the side). Side-lying leg raises is a common exercise used to strengthen the gluteus medius and is an example of abduction. Adduction is the opposite—movement towards the body's centerline. Pronation is rotating up or inward, while supination is rotating down or outward. These latter two terms often describe movement of the forearm or ankle.

17. B: Antagonists are muscles that oppose the action of the agonist (the primary muscle causing a motion). Hamstrings are the primary knee flexors (the agonists), and the quadriceps fire in opposition. The gastrocnemius does cross the knee joint, so it is a knee flexor, although secondary to the hamstrings. Tibialis anterior is on the shin and is involved in dorsiflexion.

18. A: Shoulder flexion occurs in the sagittal plane (as does most flexion from anatomical position). Shoulder flexion is bringing the arm forward up towards overhead. The sagittal plane is viewing the body from the side, dividing the body into right and left sections. Abduction and adduction occur in the frontal plane and in rotation, such as trunk twists, and typically occur in the transverse plane.

19. C: The lumbar and cervical spine both have natural lordotic curves, but the lumbar region may display pronounced lordosis beyond 60 degrees, which is deemed abnormal. Particularly with obesity prevalent in today's society, lumbar lordosis is seen more frequently. The thoracic and sacral spines display kyphotic curves.

20. C: Glycolysis is one of the anaerobic (without oxygen) metabolic pathways for producing ATP. It generates ATP from carbohydrate (glucose) metabolism that is used for two to three minutes of high intensity activity. The ATP-PC system is the other anaerobic pathway. It uses ATP stored in muscles; however, there is very little, so it is sufficient only for about ten-second high intensity bouts of activity at a time. The aerobic pathway involves the Krebs cycle. ATP is generated through the breakdown of carbohydrates and fats and, to a lesser degree, proteins. It supplies energy during long-duration endurance activities and is used when the other energy systems are depleted or insufficient, but this takes a relatively long time and would be inefficient for short bursts of energy.

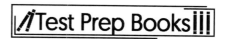

21. D: Increased submaximal heart rate is not a chronic adaptation to cardiovascular exercise; in fact, heart rate decreases at a given submaximal workload due to improvements in cardiorespiratory economy. Heart chamber size increases as does preload (the amount of blood that fills a chamber before it contracts to eject it), resulting in a higher stroke volume per heartbeat. This means that more blood, oxygen, and nutrients get moved per pump of the heart. Blood volume and hemoglobin content of the blood also increases.

22. A: DOMS typically peaks at twenty-four to seventy-two hours after exercise session completion, but may begin to develop twelve to twenty-four hours post-exercise. It is most likely to occur after high-repetition eccentric exercises, such as downhill running, as a result of microscopic damage to muscle fibers (a side effect of the repair process).

23. C: In isotonic contractions, the muscle exerts constant tension such as in a pushup or squat. Isometric contractions, like planks, are ones in which there is no change in muscle length. The body is static, and muscles are contracting to stabilize and hold the body stable against gravity. Isokinetic contractions are ones that move through the range of motion at a constant speed, but they are rarely used in practice due to the limited manufactured isokinetic equipment (some Cybex machines are isokinetic as are dynamometers). Eccentric are lengthening contractions, such as the lowering phase of a biceps curl.

24. B: Choices I, II, and IV are correct. Here are examples of correct matches:

- Fibrous: sutures in skull
- Plane: intercarpal
- Saddle: thumb
- Hinge: elbow
- Condyloid: wrist
- Pivot: radial head on ulna
- Cartilaginous: pubic symphysis

25. D: Increasing chest discomfort is a relative, not absolute, indication to terminate an exercise test. With absolute indications such as the three choices (new chest pain, cyanosis, and client's request to stop), the test must stop even if the client wants to continue, is near the end, or has not reached test termination criteria. The test may continue with relative indications so long as the client feels decent and the monitoring physician approves continuation.

26. A: RPE, or rate of perceived exertion, is a subjective measure of intensity given by the client during exercise, typically a number from six to twenty on the Borg Scale, with six being no effort and twenty indicating maximal effort. An RPE of twelve to sixteen has been shown to yield improvements in cardiovascular fitness. Because Tom is on a beta-blocker, which typically alters heart rate, the heart rate becomes an unreliable measure of exertion. Choice *B*, an RPE of fifteen to eighteen, is a greater intensity than recommended for aerobic exercise. It may be conditioning the anaerobic systems more and not be sustainable for the duration of the endurance bout.

27. D: Guidelines suggest this order, with #1 and #2 being interchangeable:
1. Skinfold
2. 1RM Bench Press
3. Push-up Test
4. Step Test
5. Sit-and-reach

The reason there are guidelines for the order of assessments is to ensure that one assessment does not affect another. Measurements of physical attributes should be first since they don't cause fatigue. Agility tests come next, though there were none listed in this practice questions. Muscular strength tests should follow, to optimize peak strength before prematurely fatiguing muscles through drawn out muscular endurance tests like the push-up test. In this case, the muscular test is the 1RM Bench Press. While there should be a rest period following this assessment, note that since it's just "One Rep Max", it won't be too tiring nor will it be aerobic. Next comes sprint tests (none here), and then local muscular endurance tests. Push-ups are a principal example of this. After muscular endurance tests, anaerobic tests and then aerobic capacity tests should be conducted. Steps tests are one of the latter. Finally, once the muscles have been given sufficient warm-up to prevent injury, flexibility tests should be performed.

28. D: Reassessment is recommended typically every four to twelve weeks, depending on the frequency of sessions, goal difficulty, and client personality. Trainers should be mindful of reassessing each component of fitness (cardiovascular, muscular strength and endurance, flexibility, and body composition), noting which areas need renewed focus and compare results to baseline. Choice *A*, every two to three weeks, is likely too short of an interval to notice progress and may result in disappointing the client and reducing motivation and satisfaction. Choices *B* and *C* are too long of a timeframe between assessments, which can also reduce motivation and thwart goal drive because it feels "too far away."

29. D: Tim is high risk because he has a known metabolic disease—the Type 1 Diabetes. The other risk factors do not even factor into his stratification because having the disease automatically makes him high risk.

30. B: Sarah has one risk factor—the smoking. Her BMI is normal. She has no known family medical history and has healthy blood pressure and blood work. She is also active.

31. C: Self-efficacy is a client's confidence in his or her ability to make a behavioral change. Self-determination is the desire to participate in an activity for one's own satisfaction, not for impressing others. Self-esteem is satisfaction in one's own worth or value, and determination is a quality that a client possesses that keeps him or her pursuing a goal or challenge, despite the work involved.

32. C: Tina has the following four risk factors: age (58 is greater than 55 years old), obesity (her BMI at 30.9 is greater than 30 kg/m^2), low HDL (< 40 mg/dL), and physical inactivity. Smoking is not a risk factor since she quit more than six months ago. Her blood pressure and fasting glucose are normal. Although her mother died of an MI, this does not count as a risk factor at age sixty-six.

33. B: The sub-scapula site is a diagonal fold on line connecting inferior angle of scapula to a point 0.8-inches from the medial border. The other three sites listed are vertical folds.

34. B: When triglycerides are greater than 150 mg/dL, it is considered a risk factor or symptom of metabolic disease. The waist circumference at 85 cm is less than the 88 cm risk factor, and the HDL at 50

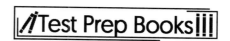

mg/dL is higher than the 40 mg/dL cutoff, which is a good thing and therefore not considered a risk factor. The fasting blood glucose is less than 100 mg/dL, so it is also normal.

35. A: Balance is the ability to control the center of mass within the base of support without falling. The wider the base of support and the lower the center of gravity, the easier it is to maintain balance. Center of gravity is the location of a theoretical point that represents the total weight of an object. Base of support is the part of an object that serves as the supporting surface, often thought of as feet in contact with the ground. The base of support also refers to the area between the feet as well, not just the physical structures of the body in contact with the supporting surface. Choice *C* is incorrect because a person cannot easily widen the center of gravity of the body. The center is a fixed point, so it can be moved, but not expanded. Choices *B* and *D* would make it harder to balance if the center of mass is raised.

36. D: If the client and trainer are not available at the same day or time to train, they are incompatible, at least until one or both schedules change. The fact that they are different sexes should have no bearing on compatibility, so Choice *B* is wrong. Choice *C* is not inherently an absolute incompatibility, especially because it states that both prefer one method (but does not indicate they cannot modify this). Choice *A* is not an issue as many clients will be less-trained or less-competitive than their trainers.

37. D: FITT-VP stands for Frequency, Intensity, Time, Type, Volume, Progression

38. B: This question requires the application of several concepts, including stratifying risk, knowing when you need a physician present during testing, and the best test selection for the goals of the patient. Paul has two risk factors for CAD: his BMI is 30.5 kg/m² (obese because > 30 kg/m²), and he takes Lipitor, which is a lipid-lowering medication. Two risk factors put him in the moderate risk stratification, where physician supervision is recommended during maximal testing and not necessary for submaximal testing. Astrand-Rhyming is a submaximal cycle ergometer test. It would be an okay choice for Paul, but because he is a runner, he is likely to have a suboptimal performance on this modality since he will experience local muscle fatigue (quadriceps). As moderate risk, Choice *D* can be ruled out because he does not need a physician present. Choice *C*, the Rockport Walk Test, is a low level test that predicts VO_2 max. It is not a very good choice for Paul because his fitness is going to be significantly higher than this test, and he likely wants a more accurate idea of his aerobic capacity. The best choice is the 1.5 mile run test, which will play to his strengths and give a great assessment of his VO_2 max, but should be physician-supervised given his risk classification. There is nothing inherently wrong with needing a physician around during testing, and the trainer should think about the goals of the client instead of the easiest option available.

Exercise Programming and Implementation

Risks and Benefits of Exercise Training and Programming for Healthy Populations

Healthy clients—including adults, seniors, children, adolescents, and pregnant women—are excellent candidates for personal training, benefitting in a number of ways. A client of any age, gender, and background can pursue personal training in order to achieve a specific goal such as fat loss, muscle gain, improved strength and endurance, improved cardiovascular and musculoskeletal systems, reduced risk of chronic disease development, or improving sports-specific skills. A qualified, knowledgeable personal trainer can minimize risks associated with exercise by designing a program for each client's individual skills, abilities, and goals, paying close attention to the client's form and execution of exercises, and closely monitoring progress to ensure that the program is challenging enough to help the client progress towards a goal, without risk of injury (or quitting) due to overworking or overloading the body unnecessarily.

Risks and Benefits of Exercise Training for Clients with Chronic Disease

Trainers will likely meet clients who have been diagnosed with a chronic disease and have received clearance from their physician to engage in beneficial physical activity. Such conditions may include stable coronary artery disease, cardiovascular diseases, diabetes mellitus, obesity, metabolic syndrome, hypertension, arthritis, chronic back pain, osteoporosis, chronic obstructive pulmonary disease (COPD), and chronic pain. Many suffering from these illnesses can benefit from cardiovascular exercise, strength training and resistance exercises, and flexibility and stretching exercises. Exercise training for clients with chronic diseases should focus on improving overall health and fitness, providing a regimen that will benefit their specific condition, and minimizing the risks of exercise. The specific health conditions of each client pose unique risks and restrictions that require different approaches for the type, duration, frequency, and intensity of exercise. Familiarity with the client's condition and awareness of limitations imposed by the condition will help the trainer design the most beneficial exercise-training program.

Health-Related Conditions to Require Medical Clearance Prior to Beginning a Program

Risk stratification is the process of classifying clients into one of three risk strata or levels (low-risk, medium-risk, or high-risk) based on the risk factors identified in the health screening process along with age, health status, and symptoms. Stratifying health concern risks is an important preliminary step in determining whether a client needs further professional medical clearance and the overall appropriateness of physical exercise, yet the personal trainer should understand that risk assessment needs to be an ongoing process. The three strata and criteria for each are as follows:

Low risk: younger (males < 45 years of age; females < 55 years), asymptomatic, and have ≤ 1 risk factor for cardiovascular or pulmonary disease

Moderate risk: older (males > 45 years of age; females >55 years) and have ≤ two risk factors for cardiovascular or pulmonary disease

High risk: diagnosed cardiovascular, pulmonary, or metabolic disease or ≥ 1 symptom of cardiovascular or pulmonary disease (e.g., dizziness or syncope, ankle edema, palpitations, pain in the chest, neck, jaw, arm, heart murmur)

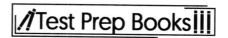

Components of Physical Fitness

Physical fitness is comprised of aspects of health that synergistically support the body's optimal functioning. Cardiovascular endurance, muscle strength and endurance, flexibility, and body composition all contribute to the body's ability to perform. Cardiovascular endurance is the ability of the cardiovascular system to pump blood throughout the body, efficiently delivering blood and essential oxygen to the muscles, tissues, and organs. Engaging in regular physical activity not only helps protect this system from conditions such as coronary artery disease, hypertension, and stroke, but also improves the functioning of all components (i.e. heart, blood vessels, arteries, etc.). Muscular strength and endurance support the skeletal system and allow for voluntary movement; exercise can improve the strength and endurance of muscles throughout the body, helping to maintain muscle mass that can deteriorate with age and sedentary lifestyles. Flexibility enables the body to perform with its full range of motion; regular flexibility and stretching exercises that keep joints mobile and muscles flexible help retain range of motion, engage in regular physical activity, and minimize injuries. Body composition refers to the relative percentages of lean mass and fat tissue. Maintaining a healthy body composition with lower body fat can minimize the risk of several illnesses.

Program Development for Specific Client Needs

Whether a client wants specific sports training, performance enhancement, lifestyle and functional training, better balance and agility, or aerobic and anaerobic improvements, an effective exercise training program incorporates a variety of physical fitness elements. A trainer must take into consideration the client's current level of fitness, their specific goals, and a realistic timeline for achieving those goals.

Sport-Specific Training

When developing an exercise training program for a client with sports-specific goals, the training regimen should focus on improving the body's endurance, strength, power, and flexibility in performing the physical movement specific to the client's sport. For example, a tennis player would benefit from exercises that improve range of motion in the upper body, core strength, agility, balance, and efficient performance of explosive movements in the legs. A swimmer would benefit from exercises focused on improving endurance and range of motion in the upper body, and the strength and power of the hip flexors.

Functional/Lifestyle Fitness

Clients focused on functional fitness benefit from a program that strengthens core muscles, improves flexibility, and increases endurance. These exercises help the client to improve their overall level of fitness, engage in regular physical activity, perform daily lifestyle activities, and minimize the risk of injury and illness. With a focus on cardiovascular exercises, regular strength training of all major muscle groups, and flexibility training, these clients will improve their overall physical and mental health.

Balance Training

Clients requiring a focus on balance and agility may be older adults, those recovering from an injury, or those with a chronic condition such as arthritis. The exercise program should have a basic routine that includes cardiovascular, strength training, and flexibility exercises to improve the client's endurance, strength, and range of motion, but also implement exercises focused on hand-eye coordination and balance. Routines that include walking up and down stairs, maintaining correct posture and form throughout a standing exercise, and engaging in regular, repetitive, low-impact cardiovascular exercises such as walking and swimming can improve the client's balance and agility in a natural progression that reduces risk of injury.

Anaerobic vs. Aerobic Training

Oxygen is required by the body when performing aerobic endurance exercises such as running, swimming, bicycling, etc., while anaerobic exercises are those that include explosive exercises performed for short durations and require little oxygen delivery to the muscles. With clients who have sports-specific goals, a training program focused on the predominant energy pathway used in their sport will improve the client's ability to perform. For example, a powerlifter would benefit from anaerobic exercise training, while a marathon runner would benefit from aerobic exercise.

Precautions and Modifications in Various Environmental Conditions

When training a client, always take environmental conditions into consideration. The client's ability to perform can be greatly affected by altitude, temperature, pollution, and environmental allergens, so keeping these effects in mind will help the client benefit from the training and safeguard them from injury or illness. At high altitudes, a client can have limited respiratory capabilities, compromised equilibrium (balance), and be at increased risk for dehydration. The trainer can implement breaks as needed and instruct the client to hydrate more frequently to minimize risks associate with altitude. In extreme temperatures and humidity, the client can experience reactions to exercise that pose serious risks. A trainer can minimize these risks by recommending moisture-absorbing/breathable clothing, closely monitoring heart rate and hydration, and implementing a longer warm-up and cool-down session. To combat environmental factors such as pollution and allergens, a trainer should move the session to an indoor location that minimizes these factors.

The Importance of Recording Exercise Sessions and Performing Periodic Reevaluations

It's imperative that trainers consistently and accurately record the client's routine, performance, and progress during every session. Not only does this allow the trainer and client to identify areas that might benefit from a different approach to training, but it also identifies areas of improvement that would benefit from increases in weight, frequency, duration, etc. By recording a client's performance each session, evaluating a client's fitness, and by adjusting the training program to continue challenging the client, the trainer is better able to fulfill their role in guiding a client to better health.

Selecting Appropriate Exercises and Training Modalities Based on Different Factors

In designing an effective exercise training, the trainer is responsible for selecting exercises and training modalities that best suit the client's abilities and restrictions. The training programs for a twelve-year-old would be far different from one for a seventy-year-old. Age impacts the recommended type, duration, and intensity of exercise. More so than age, the client's functional capacity (or training age), shown in their exercise test results, will provide the trainer with a clearer picture of a client's strengths and weaknesses. For example, clients who need to improve their flexibility would benefit from a training program implementing range of motion, strength, and endurance exercises. Those requiring improvements in strength and power might benefit from a more anaerobic-focused cardiovascular routine, with strength-training exercises using high weight and low repetitions and with less focus on flexibility.

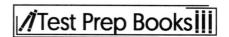

The Principles of Specificity and Program Progression

All effective exercise-training programs should consider the principles of specificity and program progression. Specificity is the focus on exercises that utilize muscle groups and functions that directly relate to a client's goals. Program progression refers to regular assessments of a client that allow a trainer to reevaluate and modify a training program to include exercises that continue to challenge the client as they increase their fitness level; in order to avoid plateaus in training, trainers should make consistent modifications to the client's exercises' frequency, intensity, duration, and type to ensure the client remains challenged and continues toward their specific goals.

Advantages, Disadvantages, and Applications of Interval, Continuous, and Circuit Training Programs for Cardiovascular Fitness

The trainer can design a workout routine that best benefits the client by applying the basics of interval, continuous, or circuit-training methods. Because each training method implements a different approach to the progression of the workout, it's best to consider the client's abilities, restrictions, and goals to determine the advantages and disadvantages of each. The trainer should remain aware of the client's program progression and improved fitness level, making adjustments as needed to ensure that the client doesn't plateau as a result of continuous training with the same method.

Interval Training

Interval training requires the client to work at a high level of exertion for brief periods with intermittent periods of rest. By challenging the cardiovascular and musculoskeletal systems to their maximal potential, providing only short rest periods, and then returning to high intensity, interval training can condition the cardiovascular system, improve endurance, and maximize metabolic functioning for improved weight loss. One benefit of interval training is that intensity is relative for each client. Therefore, with medical clearance, typically even clients with poor fitness, arthritis, or even many cardiorespiratory conditions can enjoy the variety and challenge of interval training. In these cases, trainers should keep in mind that simply walking at a faster rate, or getting up and down from a chair, may be maximum effort. Trainers should consult medical professionals if any questions arise about the safety of such workouts.

Continuous Training

Maintaining a steady speed and intensity throughout cardiovascular exercise falls into the category of continuous training. With the cardiovascular system challenged at a continuous pace for an extended duration, the benefits to the entire body include improved endurance, prolonged conditioning of muscle groups, and improved aerobic metabolic functioning. For clients who require low- to moderate-impact workouts, this mode of training can be an effective introduction to cardiovascular exercise that minimizes risk of overtraining, illness, or injury.

Circuit Training

Circuit training implements periods of cardiovascular exercise with intermittent strength training exercises. By challenging the cardiovascular system followed by musculoskeletal activities focused on muscle strength, circuit training improves cardiovascular endurance and the strength of major muscle groups that support cardiovascular function by improving the efficiency of oxygen delivery and utilization.

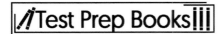

Activities of Daily Living (ADLs) in Exercise Training Program Design

While the goal of personal training is often to improve the client's overall fitness level, the client's quality of life must remain at the forefront. The trainer should be aware of the client's routine daily activities (sometimes referred to as "Activities of Daily Living" or "ADLs") and implement exercises that improve the client's abilities to perform those tasks efficiently. Trainers should consider if a client sits or stands for extended periods of time, performs repetitive motions throughout the day, utilizes upper or lower muscle groups more significantly than others, or has difficulty in the morning or afternoon hours. By knowing the client's ADLs, the trainer can tailor specific exercises to maximize benefit and improve the client's overall quality of life.

Differences Between Recommended Physical Activity and Training Principles for Different Training Goals

The ACSM guidelines for cardiovascular, strength, and flexibility training are ideal for clients seeking general fitness level improvements, but many clients will have specific training goals that require different training programs. Cardiovascular, strength, and flexibility training basics should be individually tailored by taking the client's specific goals into consideration. For example, for clients interested in weight loss, trainers would emphasize reductions in caloric intake and increases in caloric expenditure through frequent (six to seven days a week) cardiovascular, strength, and flexibility training. For clients seeking weight gain, cardiovascular activities take less priority in favor of high weight strength training coupled with increased caloric intake. Clients pursuing overall fitness improvements would benefit from a combination of cardiovascular and strength training activities. Clients focused on athletic performance enhancement require a training program that implements the principles of specificity and program progression, incorporating exercises specific to their sport.

Advanced Resistance Training Exercises

As clients progress through their exercise training program, the trainer may feel that advanced resistance training methods would improve fitness level and better achieve the target goals. With super-set training, the client is guided through repetitions of one exercise using the greatest weight that still permits proper form and then alternating with a different resistance exercise that challenges similar muscles. Olympic lifting focuses on explosive lifting of higher weights in specific defined motions (such as squat, deadlift, clean, and snatch). Olympic lifting challenges the cardiovascular and musculoskeletal systems by utilizing the anaerobic pathways. Plyometric training requires the client to perform fast repetitions of speed and power focused exercises, often with jumping and explosive movements. Pyramid training requires the client to perform exercises of high repetitions using low weight, gradually progressing to low repetitions of higher weight. While each of these advanced resistance training techniques provide cardiovascular and muscle maintenance benefits, they are often not appropriate for clients with current or previous injuries or joint-related conditions, due to the risk of further injury.

The Six Motor-Skill-Related Physical Fitness Components

In the process of training clients, the trainer should focus on the six motor skills related to physical fitness: agility, balance, coordination, reaction time, speed, and power:

Agility is a client's ability to move quickly and easily in continuous or changing directions. With exercises that require the client to maintain speed and intensity while shifting weight between opposing feet or

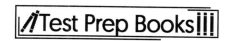

directions, a trainer can progressively improve a client's agility. Examples include short hurdles, ladder drills, and hopping in rings arranged in patterns on the ground.

Balance is a client's ability to remain steady and upright throughout the progression of an exercise. Trainers can improve a client's balance by utilizing free weights, plyometric exercises, and cardiovascular activities that strengthen core muscles.

Coordination is a client's ability to use different parts of the body simultaneously, often in different movement patterns, with efficiency and accuracy. Exercises utilizing multiple muscle groups in performing a repetitive motion or series of motions will improve this skill.

Reaction time is the time elapsed between a stimulus and a client's response. Presenting a client with a stimulus that requires a physical response can improve reaction time, which improves fitness level as well as daily tasks that require quick reactions.

Speed is the rate at which a client performs a task. Whether physically performing a single exercise or several in succession, the speed of a client's performance can serve as an easily recorded indicator of improvement in mastering specific skills and activities.

Power is a combination of force and movement, the client's ability to exert force at a given speed. Performing a sequence of exercises that require a combination of strength and mobility, a client can progressively improve their power.

Benefits, Risks, and Contraindications of Resistance Training Exercises Specific to Individual Muscle Groups

For each major muscle group, resistance-training exercises can improve strength, endurance, and metabolic function, resulting in increased fat and calorie burn. By showing clients how to perform the exercise correctly and with proper form using a suitable weight, a trainer can target specific muscle groups individually. Shoulders and arm muscles benefit from bicep curls, dips, and overhead presses. Back and chest muscles are challenged with bench presses, push-ups, flies, rows, and pull-ups. Leg and glute exercises include squats, lunges, deadlifts, and leg extensions. Abdominals respond to core-focused exercises such as crunches, leg raises, and plank exercises. Trainers must be aware of risks and contraindications inherent in these exercises, such as previous injuries that could interfere with a client's ability to perform a specific exercise correctly, pregnant women beyond their first trimester, or clients suffering from conditions related to the bones and joints.

Benefits, Risks, and Contraindications for Range of Motion Exercises

Range of motion exercises should be implemented in every exercise-training program with the goal of strengthening and stretching muscles and their related joints. Clients of all ages can suffer from limited range of motion due to lack of use, repetitive tasks, or illness or injury. A trainer can help a client improve the ability to perform exercise properly and perform daily tasks without risk of injury. Active range of motion exercises can be performed outside of formal training sessions; yoga and tai chi promote stretching in fluid motions that strengthen muscles and joints, and limit the risk of injury that can be posed by explosive or "jerky" stretching movements. Alternatively, passive range of motion exercises are those in which a force, other than the client's own strength, is used to move a joint; assistance from a partner or machines, such as in Pilates, provide the client with the force used to move the joints and muscles. Clients with injuries or existing conditions that limit mobility may benefit from passive forms of exercises, with a focus on gradually increasing range of motion.

Benefits, Risks, and Contraindications for Cardiovascular Training Exercises

Cardiovascular exercise plays an important role in improving a client's level of fitness and overall health. Because clients have unique abilities and goals, each requires a varied approach to the cardiovascular component of their exercise-training program. By considering a client's current level of fitness, experience, daily activities, skill level, and specific training goals, the trainer can design an effective cardiovascular training routine. Clients who are healthy and able to exercise regularly at moderate to high intensities can benefit from running, cycling, and swimming. Clients who have restrictive conditions such as previous injuries, chronic conditions, or even those who have previously engaged in minimal or mostly sedentary activities, should refrain from high-impact and high-intensity cardiovascular exercises, instead engaging in light- to moderate-intensity, low-impact cardiovascular exercises such as walking or swimming. Special populations such as pregnant women, those with serious health conditions, and children and adolescents can greatly benefit from cardiovascular activities specifically tailored to the individual client.

The Recommended FITT-VP for Exercise to Improve Cardiovascular and Musculoskeletal Fitness in Healthy Populations

Following the initial assessment, many clients will be deemed healthy enough to proceed with a training regimen that can be designed without special considerations given to clients with special needs. Generally, healthy adults, seniors, children, adolescents, and pregnant women who have no existing conditions of concern will be able to engage in exercise programs as follows:

Healthy adults: Prescribe an exercise program that promotes thirty to sixty minutes of cardiorespiratory activity five to seven days per week, resistance training focusing on all major muscle groups two to three days per week, and flexibility training, including stretching of major muscle groups, five to seven days per week. Cardiorespiratory activities should be performed with a target range of twelve to sixteen on the RPE scale. Strength training exercises should be performed with a focus on proper form, and stretching exercises should be held for fifteen to thirty seconds each.

Healthy seniors: Prescribe an exercise program that promotes thirty minutes of moderate physical activity five to seven days per week, and both resistance training and flexibility exercises should be incorporated five to seven days per week. While healthy seniors may not present obvious conditions of concern, it's highly recommended that the client consult a physician before engaging in more physically demanding exercise.

Healthy children and adolescents: Encourage to participate in one to two hours of age-appropriate activity daily. With a focus on individual and group sports-specific exercises, the trainer can incorporate an element of fun into the exercise training program that not only keeps the child interested, but also promotes physical fitness, endurance, agility, power, and speed for improved performance. The trainer must keep in mind that adequate hydration and frequent periods of rest during training sessions are important in ensuring the health and well-being of a child or adolescent client. Activities lasting longer than two hours should be discouraged due to heat considerations. For young children, resistance training should steer away from machines and heavier weights and focus instead on body weight exercises or use of resistance bands. This reduces the risk of injury from either improperly fitting

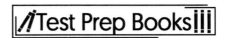

resistance machines (designed for an adult body size) or excessive weight that may injure the growing child's tissue. Proper form should always be prioritized over significant resistance.

Healthy pregnant women with no contraindications to exercise: Encourage to engage in moderate physical activity on a daily basis. For women who were sedentary prior to pregnancy, light-intensity exercises in the forms of cardiovascular activities, strength training, and flexibility should be encouraged, maintaining a focus on the client's comfort level at all times. For pregnant clients who were active prior to pregnancy, incorporating previously enjoyed activities and exercises into the exercise program will help to maintain their level of fitness throughout pregnancy, making adjustments as needed for safety concerns in each trimester (i.e. supine exercises such as supine abdominal crunches should be discouraged after the first trimester due to the possibility of reduced blood flow to the fetus). Adequate hydration and ensuring body temperature does not rise significantly should be emphasized. For this reason, exercise in hot and humid conditions may need to be modified.

The Recommended FITT-VP for Exercise Training for Clients with Chronic Disease

Some clients require special attention in developing and implementing an exercise program even after receiving medical clearance. While these general guidelines apply to clients with chronic disease, the trainer may find it necessary to make modifications as the client progresses. Constant awareness and open communication about the client's heart rate and perceived level of exertion is essential throughout each session, as are frequent breaks for hydration and rest.

Clients with stable chronic heart disease should engage in cardiovascular activity of moderate intensity for thirty minutes three to seven days per week, ideally performing five to seven hours of cardiovascular activity weekly as the client progresses in ability and endurance. Clients should perform an extended warm-up of five to ten minutes in duration prior to engaging in cardiovascular activity, and the program should also include low-impact resistance exercises two to five days per week focusing on all major muscle groups; these exercises should include five to ten exercises with one to three sets of five to fifteen repetitions. Flexibility and stretching exercises should be performed daily, with each stretch being performed two to four times, held for fifteen to thirty seconds each.

Clients with diabetes mellitus should engage in physical activity daily. Low-impact cardiovascular activities of light to moderate intensity should be performed for a duration of twenty to sixty minutes, three to four days per week; the form, intensity, and duration of the cardiovascular exercise should be prescribed in accordance with the client's abilities and comfort level in consideration. Strength training and resistance exercises should be performed three to five days per week (with forty-eight hours of rest between) and consist of one to two sets of five to twenty repetitions, focusing on each of the major muscle groups. Flexibility and stretching exercises should be performed daily, with each stretch being performed two to four times and held for fifteen to thirty seconds.

Clients with obesity should be encouraged to engage in physical activity daily. Cardiovascular exercise should be performed at a moderate intensity for forty-five to sixty minutes, five to seven days per week; these exercises should be low-impact (such as swimming or walking), gradually including a wider variety of activities and progressing in intensity as the client achieves a greater level of fitness and ability. Strength training and resistance exercises focusing on all major muscle groups should be performed three to five days per week, including five to ten exercises of fifteen to twenty-five repetitions using a moderately challenging starting weight that allows for proper form. Flexibility and stretching exercises should be performed daily, with each stretch being performed two to four times and held for fifteen to thirty seconds.

Clients with metabolic syndrome should engage in physical activity daily. Cardiovascular exercise should be performed for twenty to sixty minutes, three to four days per week, gradually increasing in frequency and intensity as the client's level of fitness and ability improves. Strength training and resistance exercises should be performed with a focus on low resistance and low intensity as the client gradually increases in strength and endurance. Programs should include one to two sets of ten to fifteen repetitions for each of the major muscle groups, increasing to fifteen to twenty repetitions as the client's program is revised. Flexibility and stretching exercises should be performed daily, with two to four stretches focusing on all the major muscle groups held for fifteen to thirty seconds each.

Clients with hypertension should engage in physical activity daily. Cardiovascular activities should be performed for thirty to sixty minutes, three to seven days per week. Strength training and resistance exercises should be performed four to seven days per week, focusing on low weight and high repetition exercises in order to avoid significant increases in systolic pressure. Flexibility and stretching exercises should be performed daily, with two to four stretches focusing on all the major muscle groups held for fifteen to thirty seconds each.

Clients with osteoporosis, chronic pain, and arthritis should engage in physical activity daily while paying attention to discomfort. If, and when, the client experiences difficulty during or following exercise, adequate rest and possible modifications should be considered before engaging in exercise again. Low-impact cardiovascular exercise should be performed at light to moderate intensity for twenty to sixty minutes, three to five days per week, gradually increasing in intensity and duration as the client's fitness and ability improve. Strength training and resistance exercises should be performed two to three days per week focusing on all major muscle groups, including one to two sets of three to twenty repetitions. Flexibility and stretching exercises should be performed daily, including two to four stretches held for fifteen to thirty seconds each.

Appropriate Exercise Modifications

Many trainers assume that modifications to exercises are only necessary when a client presents obvious limitations that interfere with their ability to perform an exercise correctly. Yet certain restrictions due to injury, limited range of motion, neuromuscular complications, and postural or physical limitations, such as scoliosis, require the trainer to tailor each exercise to the client's individual abilities and reduce the risk of injury. Even as healthy clients improve in fitness level, skill, strength, and agility, trainers should modify the existing program. The trainer's records of a client's progress over time should serve as a guide for modifications in order to continuously challenge the client and avoid plateaus. Trainers can increase resistance, decrease rest, alter the number of repetitions and sets, require more core involvement, etc. It is equally important to consider a client's intellectual level and take any impairments into account when providing instruction, education, and safety information.

Trainers can provide a variety of educational methods to clients such as newsletters, written pamphlets, posters, instructional videos, apps, and classes or seminars. The appropriateness and effectiveness of such materials may be affected by the client's age, educational level, and preference. For example, a YouTube video channel demonstrating exercises may not be appropriate for a client without internet access or an older adult who may not feel comfortable with technology. Scientific journal articles with research about fueling the body post-workout are likely not appropriate for young adolescents. Trainers can also look into community programs to recommend such as programming at the senior centers or schools.

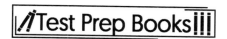

Effective Implementation of the Components of an Exercise Program

Every training session should be different, presenting the client with a variety of exercises that focus on several muscle groups, varying in frequency, intensity, duration, and type. By continuously changing these aspects of the program, the trainer ensures that the client will continue progressing in fitness level, while moving toward their ultimate fitness and health goals and avoiding plateaus, overtraining, or burnout. Using the basic components of an effective exercise training program for each session, the trainer can engage the client in a smooth progression of challenging exercises, while also addressing the client's deficits, interests, and abilities. A brief warm-up period of five to ten minutes allows a client to increase their cardiovascular activity (heart rate, respiration, blood pressure) and engage their muscles, helping the client to safely perform more rigorous activities. The main training stimulus follows the warm-up, and comprises the bulk of the workout. It should include a variety of five to ten exercises involving the cardiovascular and musculoskeletal systems. Following the training stimulus stage, the client should perform a cool-down with low-intensity activity, which permits the heart rate to return to normal, the metabolic byproducts of anaerobic respiration to be properly shuttled to the liver, and the venous blood in the extremities to be returned into systemic circulation. Stretching the major muscle groups, as well as any specific muscles targeted in the workout, should end the training session, avoiding lactic acid buildup and fatigue.

Applied Biomechanics and Exercises Associated with Movements of the Major Muscle Groups

In order to design the most effective exercise training program for each client's health and fitness goals, the trainer should be familiar with the most beneficial exercises for each major muscle group. For example, the glutes and quadriceps benefit from squats and lunges, deadlifts work the glutes and hamstrings, and calf raises target the gastrocnemius and smaller muscles on the posterior shin. Leg extensions work the quadriceps and leg curls isolate the hamstrings. Alternating these two movements can help develop balance in musculature for functional fitness. Upper bodywork should focus on muscles of the arms and shoulders, including the biceps, triceps, forearms, deltoids, and rotator cuff muscles. Exercises for these muscles include bicep curls, tricep dips or extensions, overhead presses, lateral raises, and shoulder internal and external rotation exercises. The chest and back include the pectoralis major and minor, trapezius, rhomboids, and latissimus dorsi, all of which benefit from push-ups, pull-ups, dips, and rows. The abdominals and lower back not only benefit from core exercises such as back extensions, planks, and crunches, but also from total body conditioning that keep the core engaged.

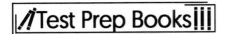

Methods for Establishing and Monitoring Levels of Exercise Intensity

Throughout a training session, the trainer should monitor the client's heart rate. This allows the trainer to determine if an exercise's intensity, load, or duration should be modified. Asking the client to report their rate of perceived exertion (RPE) on a scale of six to twenty can also be useful in determining if modifications are needed.

Borg RPE Scale

6	
7	Very, very light
8	
9	Very light
10	
11	Fairly light
12	
13	Somewhat hard
14	
15	Hard
16	
17	Very hard
18	
19	Very, very hard
20	Maximum exertion

Percentage of maximum oxygen consumption (also referred to as "VO$_2$ max") offers quantitative data to gauge intensity that can be compared to previous and future measurements in an effort to record progress. Metabolic Equivalents (METs) are another quantitative measure of exertion.

Determining Target/Training Heart Rates

In order to design the most beneficial training program, a trainer should estimate the client's maximum heart rate so that the intensity of any given activity can be calculated by measuring pulse. The trainer should be familiar with methods used to predict maximal heart rate and training heart rate goals. As research has found that maximal heart rate decreases with age, several basic formulae have been developed to predict maximum heart rate for any age. The most basic formula is simply the client's age in years subtracted from 220. For example, a forty-year-old female client's maximum heart rate (MHR) would be $220 - 40 = 180 \ bpm$.

While this formula provides a good estimate for most clients, the standard deviation is rather high, at 12 bpm, and so more precise estimation calculations have been developed. One such formula is $206.9 - (0.67 \times age \ in \ years)$.

For the same forty-year-old client, this formula yields nearly the same value, 180.1 bpm. Heart rate reserve is also used to stratify the intensity of exercise. It is calculated by recording the client's resting pulse rate and subtracting that number from the MHR. For example, a forty-year-old female with an MHR of 180 and resting pulse rate of 70, would have a 110 bpm heart rate reserve (HRR). When determining the appropriate percentage of a client's heart rate reserve, a trainer should simply multiply

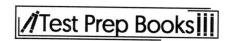

the previously determined HRR by the percentage determined appropriate for training and then add the resting pulse.

Step-By-Step

1. $220 - age = MHR$

2. $MHR - RHR\ (resting\ heart\ rate) = HRR\ (heart\ rate\ reserve)$

3. $HRR \times 0.85 + RHR = maximum\ intensity$

4. $HRR \times 0.5 + RHR = minimum\ intensity$

Example

A forty-year-old client needs to be trained at 80% of her HRR, and her resting pulse is 70. The trainer also wants to know what 50% intensity would be.

1. $220 - 40 = 180$

2. $180 - 70 = 110$

3. $110 \times 0.8 + 70 = 158$

4. $110 \times 0.5 + 70 = 125$

Clients presenting chronic conditions should train in the specific heart reserve (HRR) ranges:

- Cardiac conditions: up to 85% of HRR
- Hypertension: 40% to 70% of HRR
- Arthritis: 50% to 85% of HRR
- Diabetes: 50% to 80% of HRR
- Dyslipidemia: 40% to 70% of HRR
- Metabolic disease/obesity: initial exercise training sessions should ideally achieve 40% to 60% of HRR; as the client progresses, the target range increases from 50% to 75% of HRR.
- Osteoporosis: 40% to 70% of HRR (low- to moderate-intensity low-impact exercises)

Periodization for Cardiovascular, Resistance Training, and Conditioning Program Design and Progression

A trainer must be familiar with the concept of periodization. As a client's skills, strength, agility, balance, power, coordination, and overall fitness level improve, periods of high-intensity and low-intensity exercises can be implemented over periods of time that range from four to twelve weeks, or even one sport's season to an entire year. Routine change to the client's exercise program not only helps maintain the endurance and strength of all major muscle groups, but it also helps to reduce the risk of injury that can result from overtraining or detraining.

Determining Repetitions, Sets, Load, and Rest Periods for Specific Goals

In order to design an effective exercise-training program, a trainer must be able to determine the appropriate number of repetitions, sets, loads, and rest periods for each client. Most clients will benefit from a basic training load of 55% to 85% of their one-repetition maximum. For muscular endurance improvements, the general recommendation is for clients to perform two to three sets of fifteen repetitions or more within the weight load range of 55% to 65% of their one repetition maximum. To increase muscle size (hypertrophy), three to six sets of six to twelve repetitions at 75% of the one repetition maximum is recommended. For increases in strength, two to six sets of less than six repetitions performed at 75% to 85% of the one repetition maximum is effective. Power training would include only three to five sets of one to two repetitions performed at 90% to 100% of one repetition maximum. A rest period of two to four minutes should follow each set, with exception of power-related sets, which typically only require one minute of rest between.

Using Repetition Maximum Test Results to Determine Resistance Training Loads

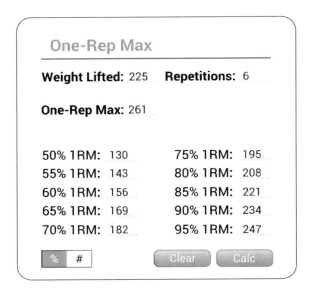

The 1 Repetition Maximum test (1RM) determines the highest amount of weight a client can safely move using the range of motion and proper form for the exercise. The test is used with both upper body and lower body strength exercises, utilizing the bench press and leg press, respectively, to help a trainer design a program that best suits the client's abilities, strengths, and weaknesses. Before performing the test, the trainer can calculate an appropriate starting test weight by multiplying the client's weight by 65 percent and using the resulting number as a starting weight. For example, a 170-pound client would start a 1RM test at 110.5 pounds (170 x .65 = 110.5).

Describing the Adaptations to Exercise Training with Regard to Strength, Functional Capacity, and Motor Skills

In developing a customized, effective exercise training program, the trainer should be able to demonstrate exercises tailored to the client for building strength, functional capacity, and improving motor skills. Resistance exercises should focus on improving muscular strength and endurance, and increasing the power and agility of major muscle groups. Functional capacity and motor skill exercises should involve all three forms of exercise (cardiovascular, strength training, and flexibility) to maximize the endurance of the cardiovascular system, the strength of major muscle groups, and the range of motion in joints.

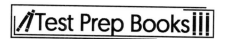

Physiological Effects and Associated Risks of the Valsalva Maneuver

The Valsalva Maneuver involves exhaling with a closed mouth and nose while exercising, typically during heavy resistance loads. The procedure can best be illustrated by describing someone pinching their nose and closing their mouth tightly while contracting the abdominal and chest muscles to exhale (often done to pop your ears mid-flight or underwater). While this maneuver has shown to effectively increase strength and power by approximately 20 percent in the performance of certain exercises, the dangers posed include limiting oxygen to the brain, causing the client to become dizzy or disoriented, and might result in the client passing out. Obviously, these risks become a major concern if the client performs an exercise with excessive weight that can lead to injury if uncontrolled. Consistent awareness of the client's breathing allows the trainer to ensure the client does not improperly use the Valsalva Maneuver in a way that poses risk of illness or injury.

Biomechanical Principles for the Performance of Common Physical Activities

Certain biomechanical principles apply to the performance of common physical activities. Running, walking, swimming, cycling, and even yoga and Pilates include movements of advancing, bending, and twisting in the frontal, transverse, and sagittal planes. By explaining each of the planes in which movement should occur, demonstrating the proper posture and techniques for performing the exercise throughout each plane, and recommending suggestions to reduce the risk of injury, a trainer can ensure the client has a thorough understanding of the exercise. It can be helpful for trainers to explain the concepts of levers, force, inertia, power, and torque in easily understandable language to give clients a basic knowledge of biomechanics.

The Concept of Detraining and Adverse Effects on Fitness and Functional Performance

"Use it or lose it" is a well-known saying. Referring to muscle mass, strength, power, and ability, this phrase sums up the concept of detraining. With injury, illness, overtraining, or quitting, clients may encounter periods in which they avoid their exercise-training program, resulting in a loss of overall fitness level and performance. Designing training programs is somewhat of an art and a science. Trainers must think critically about providing enough of a training stimulus, in the difficulty of the program, to progress clients towards goals, yet ensure the stimulus doesn't cause overloading, overtraining, or overwhelm the client so that they discontinue training. Success can be sabotaged if the program is too easy or too hard. Trainers should monitor the physical and psychological signs of overtraining or undertraining, ensuring clients remain engaged in the training program.

Signs and Symptoms of Overtraining

Clients may be overzealous in their training in anticipation of meeting goals, particularly as they begin to enjoy the benefits of an active lifestyle and experience satisfaction from reaching intermediate goals. Excessive performance of exercises can lead to overtraining and produce adverse effects in the client's training. Irritability, fatigue, disruptions in focus and mental clarity, interrupted sleep patterns, excessive muscle soreness, changes in appetite, and lack of enthusiasm in training sessions can all result from overtraining. These factors contribute to illness, injury, and discontinuation of training. In order to avoid overtraining, a trainer should emphasize the importance of rest and gradual progression throughout a training program, allowing for goals to be met without excessive physical, mental, and emotional strain.

Modifying Exercise Form to Reduce Injury

Proper technique and form throughout an exercise are imperative in ensuring the client avoids injury and reaps the most benefit. Building a strong foundation of proper form and technique for basic moves enables the client to progress to more difficult versions of the movements without the risk of injury. By modeling an exercise for a client while explaining proper form and technique, a trainer can effectively demonstrate proper performance of an exercise as well as improper techniques. By having a client repeatedly mimic an exercise as demonstrated, the trainer can ensure that the client has thorough understanding of the proper and improper actions for each exercise.

Appropriate Exercise Attire

Before commencing an exercise-training program, a trainer should discuss proper attire with a client, particularly with those who are new to being physically active. Appropriate athletic shoes should be worn for performance of cardiovascular, strength training, and flexibility exercises, enabling the client to remain balanced and comfortable. Clothing should be temperature- and exercise-appropriate with breathable layers that can be removed as a client's temperature changes, allowing for the absorption of perspiration as well. Hats and visors can also be recommended for visual comfort in outdoor activities.

Effective Communication

While training a client, effective communication is imperative. In order to effectively communicate about performance, goals, and proper form and technique, a trainer must rely on various forms of communication. Physically demonstrating and providing detailed verbal information about an exercise help to ensure that a client performs the movements correctly. Verbal and nonverbal cues before, during, and after the performance of exercises should provide the client with instruction. The client, in turn, can ask questions and demonstrate understanding of the movement through attempting the motion and talking through the form, allowing the trainer to ascertain if the client indeed understands. Asking the client open-ended questions, either verbally or in a paper questionnaire, about their experience with exercises and the program in general (whether there is difficulty, pain, comfort, or thorough comprehension) can serve as useful communication tools that allow for a client to offer feedback that they may have otherwise been uncomfortable providing. As a trainer, it's important to provide the client with a positive, nonjudgmental environment in which they feel comfortable discussing any feedback. This not only helps foster a client's satisfaction with the trainer's service, but also provides useful information that can help the trainer maintain a program design that fits the client's personal fitness and health goals.

Safely Demonstrating a Variety of Exercises

A trainer must ensure that every exercise included in a client's training program has been effectively described and demonstrated for the client. Cardiovascular activities should be modeled for the client, explaining proper form and contraindicated postures that can pose risk of injury; trainers should offer tips to minimize risk in running, walking, cycling, and swimming. Strength training routines also must be demonstrated, ideally with the client mimicking the trainer's example, to ensure that proper form and posture are maintained throughout. Range of motion exercises should be demonstrated for the client with an emphasis on the extent to which clients should stretch, the duration of each stretch, and avoidance of explosive movements.

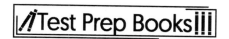

Appropriate Teaching Techniques to Demonstrate Exercises for Improving Range of Motion

Modeling range of motion exercises for the client, asking clients to mimic the exercise under the trainer's supervision, and providing verbal cues on correct posture are important teaching points to reduce injury risk and promote self-efficacy. Trainers should educate clients about the importance of full range of motion for joint health, which joints and muscles are targeted during each exercise, and how to avoid injury when performing the exercise.

Flexibility exercises can help improve range of motion, prevent injury, and prevent muscle, ligamentous, and tendon tightening. They also have a positive impact on elements of the nervous system, such as the Golgi tendon organs and mechanoreceptors, and they prepare the body to recruit the necessary motor units for optimal athletic performance. Clients should receive training on proper and improper stretching techniques and instruction to hold a position in a comfortable and moderate stretch without causing pain.

Static Stretching Exercises
Static stretches should follow the completion of the workout, especially for excessively stiff clients or those with previous injuries. Static stretching exercises can improve the muscle tension and joint relationship over time. Static stretches done prior to exercise can reduce explosive power and increase joint laxity when stiffness is required for energy conservation, placing a client at greater risk of injury.

Static stretching should take place after the workout while the muscles are warm. There is a variety of static stretches, most targeting the major muscles of the body. Some can be completed standing, such as the standing quadriceps stretch with the foot coming up behind the buttocks, stretches for the shoulders and chest, and standing hamstring and calf stretches. Seated stretches are mostly for the hips, glutes, and hamstrings. Supine stretches can be for the quadriceps, low back, and abdominals. During all static stretches, the client should be instructed to maintain good posture and joint alignment to keep joints within their normal range of motion (ROM) without hyperextension, and to keep them within their typical planes of motion (i.e., sagittal plane for flexion) without undue twisting and contorting.

Stretches are typically held at the end range of motion for 30 seconds, followed by a brief rest, then repeated for 2-3 total sets. The body should be held as still as possible, refraining from any bouncing or excessive reaching and relaxing. The joints should always be in safe, anatomically-normal positions (i.e., without hyperextending or twisting out of typical planes of motion). For example, the traditional hurdler's stretch, with one leg extended in front of the body and the other knee bent with the foot back behind the buttocks, twists the knee and can damage ligaments and is therefore contraindicated. Breathing should be smooth and steady, and clients should focus on the tension in the muscles and imagine elongating and releasing the tension.

Proprioceptive Neuromuscular Facilitation (PNF) Stretching Exercises
Proprioceptive Neuromuscular Facilitation (PNF) is a technique that uses the neuromuscular responses to specific feedback from isometric and concentric contractions performed both actively and passively. These actions and responses result in changes in the muscle/joint tension relationships and enable greater ROM to be achieved. In this way, PNF uses neurological phenomena to facilitate muscular inhibition in a specific protocol designed to improve flexibility and decrease discomfort from stretching. PNF relies on autogenic inhibition whereby inhibitory signals from the Golgi tendon organs override the excitatory impulses from the muscle spindles, resulting in gradual relaxation of the muscle. PNF is typically completed with a partner.

PNF stretching can be used for a variety of muscle groups such as the hamstrings, quadriceps, chest, and shoulder muscles. Positions vary depending on the muscle stretched. For example, hamstrings are done with the client in the supine position.

The partner or trainer must not only apply appropriate resistance for the stretching client, but also must be in the correct position, typically at the end range of the desired movement with the facilitator's shoulders and hips facing the direction of movement. How the facilitator moves directly influences how the client moves. The desired movement should bisect the facilitator's midline and center of gravity. The strength trainer's body should be positioned in such a way that the resistance applied to the client should come from the trunk and hips, not the extremities.

There are three forms of PNF stretching: hold-relax, contract-relax, and hold-relax with agonist contraction, which all begin with 10-seconds of passive pre-stretch held at the point of mild discomfort. In the hold-relax, after the pre-stretch, the partner applies a flexion force while the client holds and tries to resist the force, creating an isometric contraction for 6 seconds. The client then relaxes back into a passive stretch lasting 30 seconds, which is now a deeper stretch than the initial pre-stretch due to autogenic inhibition. Using the hamstrings as an example, in the contract-relax method after the pre-stretch, the client extends the hip while the partner resists this extension so that a concentric contraction occurs throughout the full ROM. After this, the client relaxes back into a passive hip flexion stretch of 30 seconds in duration, again deeper than initially performed due to autogenic inhibition (activation of the hamstrings, in this case). The hold-relax with the agonist contraction uses the idea of reciprocal inhibition, whereby the contraction of the agonist muscle causes relaxation of the antagonist so that after the regular hold-relax protocol, the second passive stretch is replaced with an active stretch to further increase the stretch.

Here are some examples:

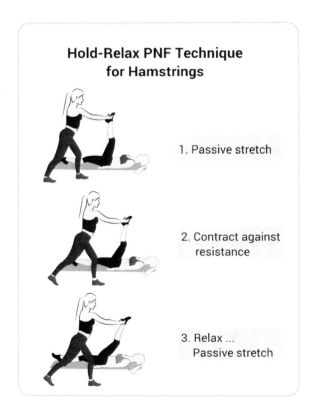

Hold-Relax PNF Technique for Hamstrings

1. Passive stretch

2. Contract against resistance

3. Relax ... Passive stretch

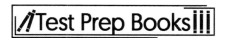

Dynamic Stretching Exercises

Dynamic stretching or mobility drills emphasize the required movements of the planned activity – rather than individual muscles – by actively moving the joint through the ROM encountered in a sport prior to the sport. Dynamic stretching occurs before the activity as part of the warm-up routine to increase heart rate, temperature, and blood flow, as well as CNS (central nervous system) and PNS (peripheral nervous system) activity to prepare the body. It promotes dynamic flexibility and mimics the movement patterns and ROM needed in sports activities without ballistic movements. It is less effective than static PNF stretching on increasing static ROM.

A neutral erect spine and athletic posture should be maintained in dynamic stretching or mobility drills. Drills such as walking lunges and hip mobility drills should use proper squatting form.

Clients typically complete 5-10 repetitions of each movement, either in place or over a given distance with a progressive increase in the ROM and/or speed on each repetition or set. The movement mechanics of the sport should be reinforced in the mobility drill, along with the predominant joint positions, such as ankle dorsiflexion on a high knee drill for sprinters.

Safely Demonstrating Various Resistance-Training Modalities

As a client progresses in their exercise-training program, the trainer can implement more advanced modalities of resistance training. Specialized equipment such as kettlebells, TRX straps, and medicine balls, as well as external and static resistance devices, add a variety of resistance training modalities to a challenging exercise program. Using different equipment and exercises can help clients improve fitness level, strength, and power, while preventing boredom, burnout, and injury. Trainers should repeatedly demonstrate proper form and technique, providing detailed descriptions of the exercise's goals and common mistakes that pose risk of injury. Spotting and consistently providing verbal and nonverbal cues will help to ensure that the client masters the techniques and performance of exercises.

Dumbbells and barbells are the most commonly used free weight training equipment. While both involve "lifting weights," this equipment differs from resistance machines in that weight plates, dumbbells, and barbells are used in varying weights for any number of exercises being typically held in the hands of the client.

Resistance machines typically enable the proper form to be achieved more easily for exercises because they only allow movement in certain planes of motion based on the mechanical setup of the levers, hinges, pulleys, and movable pieces. However, this guidance, restriction, and stabilization make exercises completed on resistance machines less sports-specific than free weights, plyometric, or body weight exercises in which the client must stabilize the body while moving through the range of motion. Weight machines can be a good starting place for beginners and also for senior clients and others who have poor balance and coordination, and for certain exercises for individuals recovering from injuries. This is because these machines are generally safer to use and usually only isolate one movement, which makes them easier to use and a good way for beginners to grasp one specific movement at a time. Resistance machines can be helpful for rehabilitating certain body parts because they generally isolate a specific muscle group. In general, this is not advantageous for overall strength-training, especially for sports-specific work important to competitive clients. However, resistance machines have their place, particularly in injury rehab, solo sessions, rapid circuit training, and reaching higher maximal lifts. For heavy weights and maximal efforts, most machines have the advantage of not requiring a spotter, although clients should still always exercise caution when attempting any lift. Some machines force the correct movement for the lift, which may help reduce the risk of injury and ensure that the client is moving through the entire range of motion for each repetition. Machine workouts can be more efficient because they are generally organized in a circuit in the layout of the gym, so the client can easily move from one to another. With that said, if clients prioritize saving time and they do not properly adjust the settings to fit the machine to their body, clients can "cheat" in the movement and increase injury risk.

Most weight machines require the client to move the weight in a predetermined path, making it difficult to strengthen the stabilizer muscles. Similarly, usually only one exercise can be completed on each machine, making it cumbersome to keep getting up, moving to another machine, and adjusting the settings accordingly. Most machines are designed for the average-sized adult, so small youth clients, slight women, or significantly taller and larger clients may find the fit less than ideal, even when adjusted as much as possible, resulting in a fit that is not only uncomfortable, but may cause difficulty performing the exercise correctly.

Safely Demonstrating Various Functional Training Exercises

As a client's range of motion improves, modifications can be made to their exercise-training program to include a variety of functional training exercises. To ensure a client's safety and their ability to use equipment such as resistance bands, stability balls, balance boards, foam rollers, and medicine balls, the trainer must provide a thorough demonstration and carefully observe the client's performance of each exercise. Not only will this maximize the physiologic benefits and reduce risk of injury, but it will also help to improve the client's ability to master technique and form, allowing for the implementation of increasingly more challenging exercises.

Proper form is especially important during high-intensity activities when muscles, joints, tendons, and ligaments are under very high loads and speeds, subjecting them to increased force and demanding power. Trainers should instruct clients to land all jumps with soft and slightly flexed knees, to pump arms powerfully and efficiently, and to breathe as much as possible. Even though these activities are not consuming a significant amount of oxygen due to their intensity and reliance on anaerobic metabolism, focusing on adequate breathing helps to maintain proper form and assists in a more rapid and comfortable recovery to quickly oxygenate the muscles and metabolic byproducts of anaerobic metabolism. When running stairs or uphill sprints, clients should lift knees as high as possible. They should maintain a slight forward lean from the ankles and not the waist, and use aggressive, powerful arm swings. When descending, steps should be light and quick. Slight knee flexion will help protect knee cartilage and ligaments. Some clients might choose to walk down hills backwards or otherwise mix up the downhill routine.

Heavy battle ropes are a great training tool for a total body workout, upper body power, endurance, and anaerobic bouts. There is a wide variety of exercises and patterns that can be implemented. A proper athletic stance should be encouraged, with the good squatting form of knees flexed, hips staying back behind the ankles, erect spine, good posture, chest up and out, and eyes forward. Most anaerobic activities are short enough in duration that clients should be able to maintain mental focus on sustaining intensity and using good form throughout the duration. Trainers should provide adequate recovery between bouts of heavy exertion to ensure that clients are able to truly maximize their efforts on each attempt.

Proper Spotting Positions and Techniques

Spotting procedures help clients complete exercises safely and efficiently. Not only do trainers need to know how to execute correct spotting techniques, but they must be able to demonstrate and teach the

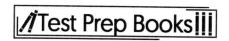

techniques to clients so that they can spot one another during partner activities. Spotting also helps monitor a client's lifting form and movement execution, allowing the spotter to give verbal cues and help correct any errors in execution. It also allows for motivation, instruction, encouragement, feedback, and certain exercise modifications that would otherwise not only be dangerous, but physically impossible, without spotters. An example is negative resistance training, wherein clients can handle greater weight on the eccentric or lowering portion, but need spotters to help raise the weight in the concentric phase. Spotters should be prepared to offer as much help as needed. Clear communication between the lifter and spotter is required for safety, and the pair should discuss the lift before it occurs. The spotter should ensure that the weights are evenly spaced and equally loaded on the bar and that the collars are properly used.

Number of Spotters Needed for Given Situations and Exercises

The required number of spotters is determined by the load being lifted, the experience and skill of the client and spotters, and the physical strength of the spotters. The spotters must be strong enough to handle the load that the client is lifting with little notice and sometimes in less than ideal angles and positions. Therefore, it is crucial that spotters are honest with themselves and lifters about their abilities. It is better to err on the side of caution and use multiple spotters when necessary, as long as they can be accommodated spatially around the lift without being overly cumbersome. With the exception of power exercises, free weight exercises should use a minimum of one or two spotters when a client moves the bar over the head or face, or has it on the front of the shoulders or positioned on the back during the execution. During power exercises, clients should be instructed to push the bar away or drop it when the bar is in front, and release it or jump forward when the bar is missed behind the head. A spotter should not be used. Two spotters are sometimes needed with heavy lifts, especially bar lifts, where one spotter should be at each end of the bar.

Spotter Location

The location of the spotter or spotters depends on the lift being attempted. For exercises with heavy weights on a bar such as a front squat, often two spotters are needed at each end of the bar to help balance the weight with the athlete and lift from either side, should an issue occur. For standing exercises such as squats and deadlifts, spotters should stand behind the lifter while the bar is still on the rack and as the lifter gets into position. They should then move as close as possible toward the lifter without touching him or her, as the lifter steps away from the rack with the bar. The spotter's hands should be in the ready position near the bar while the lifter raises and lowers the weight. Once the set is complete or when failure is indicated by the lifter, the spotter should assist the lifter in returning the bar to the rack by holding onto the bar and guiding it back to the racked position. During exercises such as a dumbbell bench press, spotters should keep their hands near the lifter's forearms, close to the wrists. For a seated overhead triceps extension with a barbell, spotters should straddle the flat bench.

Body and Limb Placement Required When Spotting the Lifter

Once the spotter and the lifter are in the correct positions, the spotter needs to pay attention to their body and limb placement for their own safety during the lift as well as that of the client. When spotting over-the-face barbell exercises, the spotter should grasp the bar with an alternated grip, usually narrower than that of the athlete's grip. The spotter also should use a solid, wide base of support and a neutral spine position. Spotters should use an athletic stance, with feet slightly wider than hip-width apart, knees flexed, arms and hands up and in a ready position that is close to the bar and athlete without touching them. Bodyweight should be equally and soundly distributed on both feet, which should be firmly planted on the ground. Spotters must follow the movement of the client and the bar with their eyes as well as their hands, and remain intensely focused on the task at hand until the bar is

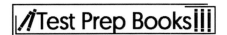

re-racked. Spotters and lifters should communicate throughout the lift if anything changes, but it is the spotter's job to verbally motivate and check in with the lifter, since the client is likely less physically and mentally able to talk during maximal exertion.

Normal and Abnormal Responses to Exercise and Criteria for Termination of Exercise

Throughout the exercise-training program, a trainer must be constantly aware of the client's response to exercise, closely monitoring the physical cues that indicate normal and abnormal responses to activity. In the beginning stages of training, while fitness levels are lower, clients may have elevated heart rates, excessive perspiration, labored breathing, and signs of fatigue early in the session, depending on their baseline level of fitness. While these physical responses are normal, a trainer should provide clients with adequate rest periods, allow for frequent hydration, and closely monitor a client for verbal and nonverbal cues of excessive distress, such as sudden onset of chest or arm pain, headache, and dizziness. If warning signs appear, a trainer should allow the client to rest until their physical state returns to normal. If serious warning signs continue, a trainer should seek medical attention immediately and instruct the client to provide medical clearance to continue exercise from their physician. It's prudent to use rate of perceived exertion during the first few weeks of training as an important adjunct to any physiological signs of intensity. If the client feels as though he or she is working really hard, the intensity may need to be dialed back.

Proper and Improper Form and Technique While Using Cardiovascular Conditioning Equipment

Indoor cardiovascular training equipment such as treadmills, elliptical machines, stationary bicycles, and stair-climbers provide clients and trainers with all-weather activities that can be performed at a pre-selected intensity and duration. For these modes of training to be optimally effective with minimal risk of injury, trainers should instruct clients on proper form and technique as well as educate clients on the necessary use of emergency stop buttons. While remaining upright, well-balanced, and able to perform the activity without leaning on the machine, the client should be monitored by the trainer throughout the exercise—at least initially during the learning stage—to ensure that the client's form and technique remain consistent. Leaning or relying on the handrails may indicate that the level of the machine or the speed is too rigorous for the client.

Trainers can make use of a variety of cardiovascular machines such as treadmills, bicycles, rowing machines, stair steppers, elliptical trainers, arm ergometers, and Arc trainers. The choice of the equipment may depend on the client's sport, training goals, availability, preference, injury, and workout plan. Trainers should teach clients how to use the console, properly program the machine with the various inputs, and the proper form for each piece of equipment. For example, it is a common mistake to set an improper seat height on spin bikes and stationary bikes, often resulting in a seat that is too low, a knee that is too flexed, and a less-efficient stride. Clients should set the seat height so that they fully extend their knee and straighten the leg downward. From there, they should lower the seat so that there is about 10 degrees of knee flexion at the lowest point in the cycle rotation.

Clients should use normal, healthy posture whether seated or standing and refrain from leaning on handrails. The spine should be in optimal alignment, with shoulders back and chest open. Clients should avoid reading or watching video if it compromises form or causes slouching. On elliptical machines that include arm pedals, the elbows should be flexed to roughly 90 degrees, hands should have a neutral grip, and shoulders should remain relaxed. A recumbent bike can be used when the torso needs

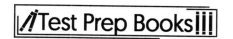

significant support; for example, in cases of upper extremity injury or rib fracture. However, in terms of cardiovascular benefit, this machine typically falls significantly short of other modes. On all cycle types, clients should keep their torso upright and refrain from oscillating from side to side with each alternating pedal stroke. Pedal rate should typically mimic that of running at about 90 revolutions per minute, unless the client is specifically working on turnover, in which case the resistance can be lowered and over-speed training can occur. Some bikes display metabolic equivalents (METs), which serve as an indication of energy expenditure over that at rest and can be used as a gauge of intensity. Resistance coupled with speed factor into bicycling METs, while body weight, incline, and speed (pace) influence metabolic equivalents during treadmill running. An arm ergometer can be a good choice in cases of severe lower extremity injury or disability, or for clients who need to work on upper body strength and muscular endurance, such as gymnasts and swimmers. This machine involves sitting upright in the provided chair and pedaling with the arms, much in the same way a normal bicycle functions with the legs.

Proper and Improper Form and Technique While Performing Resistance Exercises

During resistance training exercises, trainers should closely monitor the client's form. With plyometric activities, as well as those involving free weights, stability balls, etc., a client's focus should remain on continuously maintaining proper form throughout the exercise. Not only does proper form and technique allow for the exercise to target the intended muscle groups, but they also reduce the risk of compromising muscles and musculoskeletal structures not intended to be involved in the exercise. Until a client has mastered the performance of a strength training exercise, a trainer should closely monitor and correct a client's performance of the entire activity.

The proper execution of lifting exercises with free weights should be demonstrated and explained thoroughly by strength trainers. Clients often have different learning styles, so the execution and explanation of proper form and technique in exercises is imperative to convey this information to each client. Each exercise obviously has its own set of procedures for proper execution, but in general, emphasis on form and breathing technique will lead to successful execution. With exercises that are completed in a standing position, knees should be slightly relaxed and not locked, feet should be facing forward, and a strong core should be engaged to support the erect spine. Exercises in the seated and supine positions require five points of contact for optimal body support: the head is firmly on the bench or back pad, the shoulders and upper back are evenly placed and firmly on the bench or back pad, the buttocks are positioned evenly on the bench or seat, and the right and left foot are both placed flat on the floor.

In American society today, daily activities tend to focus on forward posture such as typing on a computer or holding a cell phone in front of the face and hunching over to type on it. This chronic slouched posture can lead to tightness in the anterior muscles of the chest and a stretching and weakening of posterior muscles of the shoulders, neck, and upper back. Trainers often need to remind clients to pull their shoulders back and engage their rhomboids and keep their chest up and out, which opens it up for both improved breathing mechanics and a healthy posture. In all standing exercises, swinging the weights should be avoided, and clients should attempt to hold their bodies as still in the upright position as possible, refraining from swaying and rocking, which uses momentum to augment the lifting motion. Clients should be instructed to exhale, mostly through the mouth, during the concentric or more challenging lifting portion of the movement through the sticking point (the hardest point of the exercise). They should then inhale slowly through the nose during the eccentric or easier phase, depending on the motion.

In most cases, holding the breath such as in the Valsalva maneuver is contraindicated, and it can greatly increase blood pressure and cause dizziness and disorientation. However, it can be used in certain core exercises with care as a way to increase torso rigidity and aid support of the vertebral column. This lessens compressive forces on the intervertebral discs and supports the normal and neutral lordotic lumbar spine. These same benefits can be achieved through the use of a weight belt, which should be used for exercises that stress the lower back, especially at near maximal loads.

With the exception of power exercises, free weight exercises should use a minimum of one or two spotters when a client moves the bar over the head or face, has it on the front of the shoulders, or positioned on the back during the execution. When performing an incline bench press, the weight bar should make contact with the upper chest at the sticking point. In contrast, with a flat or decline bench press, the bar should make contact slightly lower – at or below nipple line. Proper form with a good neutral erect spine, chest up and out, feet flat on the floor, and shoulders back should be used on resistance machines. The height of the bench or chair portion can usually be adjusted and should be so that the knees are flexed to 90 degrees and the feet are flat on the floor. For machines such as the leg press, the feet should be placed on the platform slightly wider than hip-width. Knees should flex in alignment with the ankles, refraining from any tendency to deviate them laterally, which internally rotates the hips and places undo stress on the lateral compartment of the knee. Hand grip should be neutral and evenly spaced in most cases, unless a narrow or wide grip is specifically introduced as a modification. Most machines have pictures of proper alignment and positioning of pads and bars so that clients can adjust the machine to fit their bodies. Clients should align their joint axes with the axis of rotation of the machine to optimize joint function and prevent any incongruity in the moving axes, which can induce injury.

Proper and Improper Form and Technique for Flexibility Exercises

In teaching range of motion exercises, the trainer should inform the client of the specific muscle groups targeted, the extent and duration to which a stretch should be held, and provide tips to recognize signs of overstretching beyond physical limitations. Quick, ballistic movements should be contraindicated, and partner-assisted stretching should be done within a pain-free range of motion at all times.

Interpreting Client Understanding During Exercise

An observant trainer will become familiar with each client's verbal and nonverbal cues, indicating the client thoroughly understands procedures. After the trainer explains and demonstrates an exercise, a client may present verbal cues such as questions that indicate further explanation and demonstration may be necessary. Nonverbal cues such as improper form and technique or even quizzical looks, sighing, and sounds of frustration also indicate that the client has not yet grasped the exercise.

Effective Communication and Feedback

It is important for trainers to be effective communicators and active listeners. Verbal and nonverbal behaviors are equally important in setting a positive, educational, and supportive environment for the client. The trainer should follow these behaviors:

- Look professional and fully attentive
- Give eye contact
- Use encouraging facial expressions and body language
- Augment interaction with positive verbal feedback, demonstrations, instructions, and cueing

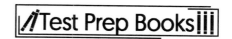

Body language such as hands on hips or crossed over the chest may appear standoffish. Conversely, smiling and nodding enhance client comfort and satisfaction. The trainer should refrain from checking phone messages, complaining about his or her life, or acting distracted in any number of ways.

Specific Exercises and Program Modifications for Healthy Populations

Generally healthy clients, with minimal health concerns, benefit from an exercise training program that includes a variety of cardiovascular, strength training, and flexibility exercises. Throughout the progression of a training program, clients may require modifications that ensure the elements of their program continue to support their goals. Modifications to increase the frequency, intensity, time, and type (FITT) of a client's program should be made regularly in accordance with periodic assessments. Pregnant women who regularly engage in exercise, and wish to continue their training throughout the pregnancy, should have modifications made to particular exercises that put pressure or strain on the core; exercises performed in the supine position should be modified to take place in a semi-recumbent position after the first trimester to protect the health and safety of both the mother and fetus.

Specific Exercises and Program Modifications for Individuals with Chronic Disease

Trainers will work with clients who have been medically cleared for exercise, but who also struggle with chronic health conditions affecting the cardiovascular, musculoskeletal, or neuromuscular systems. These clients benefit from regular cardiovascular, strength training, and flexibility exercises, and should participate in a training program designed with their particular health condition in mind. Taking care to identify the restrictions associated with a client's condition, a trainer can design an effective training program that improves a client's health, while minimizing risk of illness or injury. Still, the program must also provide a sufficient challenge to cause physical health improvements. Assessments should be performed more frequently with clients with chronic illness to make sure that the exercises included in their training programs are appropriate in frequency, intensity, type, and duration at a gradual, healthy pace.

Principles of Progressive Overload, Specificity, and Program Progression

All exercise training programs should be designed based on a client's fitness and health goals, taking into account all components of health-related fitness as well as areas of greatest deficit. Then, progressive overload, specificity, and program progression should be determined in order to plan a program that will help a client work towards their goals. When modifying a client's program following regular assessments that help a trainer determine when a client has progressed to a point where frequency, intensity, duration, or type of exercises should increase, trainers should consider progressive overload. Not only does appropriate program progression ensure that the client remains challenged and on track toward their goals, but it also minimizes the chance of plateauing in a program that is too consistent and lacks sufficient training stimulus.

Appropriate Methods to Teach Progression of Exercises for All Major Muscle Groups

To ensure that a client's training program follows a consistent progression, a trainer can implement modifications to exercises. As a client masters an exercise, trainers should try incremental increases in resistance and progress to more challenging forms of exercises. Lower body exercises can progress from a standing squat to a stationary lunge to walking lunge. Upper body exercises can increase in intensity by adding resistance (weights, bands, etc.) and by increasing the range of motion. Core exercises can

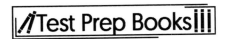

increase in number of sets and repetitions and follow more advanced techniques, such as bending and twisting while maintaining proper form.

Modifications to Periodized Conditioning Programs

Periodized training programs consist of specific periods of time designated to focus on specific skills, strengths, or abilities, which are later modified in the next period to address new skills or another area of focus. For example, the first period of an athlete's periodized program might focus on strength and power, the second on agility and speed, the third on mastering motor skills and coordination, and the last might address specific exercises that develop skills unique to the client's specific sport. While these periodized portions of the program should have specific areas of focus, a trainer should ensure that the client continues to perform and progress with exercises focused on cardiovascular, strength training, and flexibility simultaneously. Not only does this method ensure that the client improves fitness level and overall health, but it also helps to avoid plateaus or deconditioning effects.

Effective Techniques for Program Evaluation and Client Satisfaction

A trainer should consistently seek feedback from clients not only to ensure satisfaction but also gauge the client's physical and psychological state at various points throughout the program to prevent injury, boredom, and burnout. Before, during, and following training sessions, a trainer should ask clients to assess their progress, their enjoyment of the exercises and program in general, and ask any specific questions about aspects of their training program. Trainers should provide a client with surveys or some other assessment of their satisfaction to determine if changes should be made to better serve the client and support their ultimate success.

Client Goals and Appropriate Review and Modification

In the initial consultation and assessment, the trainer and client should establish the baseline, which is the client's beginning fitness level, skill, and ability. From there, the trainer and client should work together to determine reasonable objectives and S.M.A.R.T. goals for training, outline the fitness level, skills, and abilities associated with those goals, and develop an appropriate exercise training program that gradually progresses a client from baseline to their goals. As clients master skills and improve at different rates throughout training, it's imperative that a trainer consistently reviews a client's performance and modifies a training program's elements accordingly. By providing the client with regular assessments, requesting a client's feedback, and implementing modifications that continuously challenge a client and support their progress, a trainer can ensure that a client is satisfied and successful.

Practice Questions

1. What does specificity refer to?
    a. The flow of a training program's specific sessions
    b. The specific goals of the client
    c. Exercises for muscle groups related to a client's specific goal
    d. A client's specific statistics (age, weight, etc.)

2. What does program progression refer to?
    a. A client's overall progress
    b. Modifications to ensure a client progresses
    c. A client's perception of progress
    d. Progression in a client's age

3. Which of the following is true regarding a client's medical history?
    a. It should not be considered
    b. It should be discussed thoroughly
    c. It does not indicate illness or injury
    d. It is not necessary for program planning

4. What does interval training refer to?
    a. Sessions performed indoors or outdoors
    b. Discontinuing workouts after the warm-up and cardiovascular component
    c. Maintaining steady speed throughout the workout
    d. Changing speed and intensity of workouts during a session

5. What does continuous training refer to?
    a. Performing the same workout for the entire duration of the session
    b. Engaging in the same workout every session throughout the training program
    c. Maintaining a steady speed throughout a cardiovascular exercise
    d. Continuing from one exercise to the next without rest

6. What does circuit training refer to?
    a. Engaging in indoor or outdoor activities only
    b. Allotting one specific exercise focus per session
    c. Using a combination of cardiovascular and strength training exercises
    d. Working all major muscle groups in one session

7. Which of the following is true regarding activities of daily living?
    a. They are not important for program design
    b. They should be performed outdoors
    c. They should be practiced in sessions
    d. They should be considered when designing a training plan for a client

8. For weight loss, recommendations include all EXCEPT which of the following?
    a. Frequent cardiovascular activity
    b. Increased caloric intake
    c. Higher number of resistance training sets
    d. Increased frequency of flexibility training

9. Regarding athletic performance enhancement, which of the following statements is true?
   a. Sports-specific activities should be included in training
   b. Only major muscle groups involved in the specific sport should be the focus
   c. Diet does not need to be considered
   d. Sessions do not require warm-up or cool-down periods

10. Which of the following statements is true about advanced resistance training exercises?
    a. They should only be recommended for weightlifters
    b. They should not be performed by seniors
    c. They require clients to have progressed to a certain level of fitness first
    d. They include swimming, cycling, and running

11. Which of the following statements is true about plyometric training?
    a. It uses machines primarily
    b. It includes box jumps and bounding drills
    c. It is contraindicated for pregnant women
    d. It should be used only in programs for advanced clients

12. Which of the following statements is true about pyramid training?
    a. It focuses on clients' skills in gymnastics
    b. It requires a client to be in the supine position throughout the training session
    c. It uses only leg muscles
    d. It includes high reps of low weight progressing to low reps of high weight

13. The six motor skills related to physical fitness include all EXCEPT which of the following?
    a. Creativity
    b. Agility
    c. Power
    d. Balance

14. What is the bench press an example of?
    a. A cardiovascular exercise
    b. A chest exercise
    c. A range of motion exercise
    d. An advanced exercise contraindicated for healthy seniors

15. What is the plank exercise an example of?
    a. An exclusively outdoor exercise
    b. A swimming exercise
    c. An abdominal and core exercise
    d. An exercise not recommended for children and adolescents

16. When should pregnant women consider modifying the exercise?
    a. Before eating
    b. After eating
    c. After the first trimester
    d. Only in exercises focused on abdominals and legs

17. Which of the following statements is true about range of motion exercises?
    a. They are only necessary for seniors
    b. They should never be performed by cardiac patients
    c. They should be included in all training programs
    d. They should be performed twice weekly

18. Which of the following statements is true about cardiovascular exercises?
    a. They include swimming, running, and cycling
    b. They include stretching specific joints
    c. They are contraindicated for children and adolescents
    d. They should only be performed outdoors

19. Which of the following statements is true about strength training exercises?
    a. They can be performed with body weight or external resistance modalities
    b. They include swimming, running, and cycling
    c. They are contraindicated for pregnant women
    d. They should only include exercises using machines

20. Which of the following is true for healthy populations?
    a. They require medical clearance for exercise
    b. They do not require monitoring of exertion during exercise
    c. They do not require rest or hydration during sessions
    d. They should incorporate cardiovascular, resistance training, and flexibility in their programs

21. Trainers should follow which of the following guidelines for clients with chronic conditions?
    a. They should not engage in any cardiovascular activities
    b. They should avoid range of motion exercises
    c. They should follow a low-calorie diet
    d. They should incorporate low- to moderate-impact activities in their program

22. Which of the following is true for clients with arthritis and osteoporosis?
    a. They benefit from low-impact cardiovascular exercise
    b. They should adhere to major dietary restrictions
    c. They frequently miss training sessions
    d. They should not perform outdoor cardiovascular exercise

23. Which of the following guidelines is true regarding obese clients?
    a. They should not perform range of motion exercises
    b. They should not perform strength-training exercises for the legs
    c. They should avoid planking and abdominal crunches
    d. They should perform cardiovascular activity five to seven days per week

24. The proper flow of activities in a training session looks most like which of the following?
    a. Stretching, strength training, cool-down, cardiovascular
    b. Warm-up, training, cool-down, stretching
    c. Warm-up, stretching, cool-down, strength training
    d. Cardiovascular, stretching, warm-up, cool-down

25. Effective methods of monitoring exercise intensity include all EXCEPT which of the following?
    a. The Valsalva Maneuver (VM)
    b. Rated-perceived exertion (RPE)
    c. Maximum oxygen consumption (VO$_2$ max)
    d. Metabolic equivalents (METs)

26. The arms and shoulders include all muscles EXCEPT which of the following?
    a. Hamstrings
    b. Biceps
    c. Triceps
    d. Forearms

27. The legs include all muscles EXCEPT which of the following?
    a. Hamstrings
    b. Quadriceps
    c. Calves
    d. Deltoids

28. The chest and back include all muscles EXCEPT which of the following?
    a. Hamstrings
    b. Deltoids
    c. Trapezius
    d. Pectoralis Major

29. What does the Borg RPE Scale determine?
    a. A client's weight classification on a scale of six to twenty
    b. A client's preference of cardiovascular activity
    c. A client's heart rate on a scale of one to one hundred
    d. A client's exertion on a scale of six to twenty

30. The Karvonen method considers which aspects of a client?
    a. Weight and height
    b. One rep maximum (1RM) and age
    c. Age and pulse rate
    d. Pulse rate and 1RM

31. What does periodization refer to?
    a. A client's schedule of sessions
    b. The frequency of range of motion exercises
    c. The intensity levels of exercises per period or cycle of training
    d. A rest period schedule per session

32. Healthy clients should have an initial basic training load of?
    a. 55% to 85% of 1RM
    b. 10% to 25% of 1RM
    c. 90% to 100% of 1RM
    d. 15% of 1RM

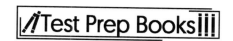

33. For endurance, clients should perform two to three sets of which of the following?
    a. Fifty or more reps
    b. Fifteen or more reps
    c. Two to three reps
    d. One rep at 1RM

34. For muscle mass gain, clients should perform three to six sets of which of the following?
    a. Six to twelve reps
    b. Fifteen to twenty-five reps
    c. Fifty or more reps
    d. One to two reps at 1RM

35. Components of physical fitness include all EXCEPT which of the following?
    a. Endurance
    b. Hygiene
    c. Flexibility
    d. Body composition

36. Training with focus on specific muscles and skills associated with specific sports would be an example of which of the following?
    a. Interval training
    b. Periodized training
    c. Sports-specific training
    d. Resistance training

37. Training programs implementing short exercises requiring little or no oxygen would be classified as which of the following?
    a. Anaerobic
    b. Aerobic
    c. Cardiovascular
    d. Range of motion

38. Training programs implementing endurance activities requiring oxygen would be classified as which of the following?
    a. Anaerobic
    b. Aerobic
    c. Power-lifting
    d. One Repetition Maximum

39. If a client reports new-onset discomfort in the chest and arms, the appropriate action of the trainer would be to?
    a. Continue exercise for the full session
    b. Seek medical assistance
    c. Call the client's physician
    d. Send the client home

40. Training clients at higher altitudes can result in which of the following?
    a. Dehydration
    b. Improved performance
    c. Increased leg strength
    d. Elation

41. The FITT-VP principle includes all EXCEPT which of the following?
    a. Frequency
    b. Teachability
    c. Time
    d. Type

42. Which of the following factors would NOT affect a client's ability to increase his or her training load?
    a. Lack of sleep
    b. Poor diet
    c. Training too often
    d. Focusing on core exercises

43. Which physiological adaptation is expected after a client has participated in an aerobic-training program?
    a. Heart rate reserve decreases and resting-heart rate increases
    b. Heart rate reserve increases and resting-heart rate decreases
    c. Heart rate reserve increases and resting-heart rate increases
    d. Heart rate reserve decreases and resting-heart rate decreases

44. Which of the following statements about rest periods is NOT true?
    a. Longer rest periods promote nervous-system recovery
    b. Longer rest periods promote muscular-system recovery
    c. Longer rest periods promote cardiovascular conditioning
    d. Shorter rest periods promote cardiovascular conditioning

45. A client wants to increase muscular hypertrophy for a bodybuilding competition. How many repetitions and exercises should be assigned to optimize success in the stated goal?
    a. Six to twelve repetitions per set; three exercises per muscle group
    b. Two to four repetitions per set; three exercises per muscle group
    c. Fifteen repetitions per set; three exercises per muscle group
    d. Six to twelve repetitions per set; one exercise per muscle group

46. Which of the following is true regarding muscle balance?
    a. The strength in opposing muscle groups must be equalized.
    b. The strength ratios in antagonist muscle groups must be improved.
    c. Muscle balance is not an integral part of a strength-training program.
    d. Even if a client has improper muscle balance, the body will maintain its normal movement patterns during exercises.

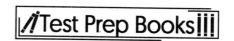

47. Which type of exercises give muscle tissue the most stimulation and are beneficial for limited training time and which type of exercises involve the core muscles and should be the basis of training programs?
  a. Multi-joint; Assistance
  b. Structural; Primary
  c. Primary; Assistance
  d. Multi-joint; Structural

48. A client has limited time to train. She wants to improve mental focus and lose body fat. Which type of training would benefit her most?
  a. Split-routine training
  b. 1RM
  c. Circuit training
  d. Percentage-based training

49. A client would like to improve strength and power for a weightlifting competition. In which order should she complete the following exercises?
    I. Olympic lifts
    II. Back extensions
    III. Bicep curls

  a. I, II, III
  b. II, I, III
  c. III, II, I
  d. II, III, I

50. How many repetitions and sets should be used when training a client for muscular endurance?
  a. Six to twelve repetitions for three sets
  b. Six to twelve repetitions for five sets
  c. Twelve to fifteen repetitions for three sets
  d. Two to six repetitions for five sets

51. Which of the following is NOT an appropriate progression method for promoting physiological adaptations in a client during the training phase?
  a. Increasing training-load intensities to improve speed
  b. Increasing training density
  c. Increasing training volume
  d. Changing the duration of rest between sets

52. Which of the following approaches should be used to help a client recover from previous training sessions and improve neural patterns while promoting supercompensation?
  a. Linear periodization
  b. Unloading/deloading week
  c. Undulating/nonlinear periodization
  d. Rehabilitation

53. Which of the following exercises would help a client restore neuromuscular control after an injury?
    a. Doing bodyweight squats on a flat surface
    b. Jumping on a flat surface
    c. Doing push-ups on a flat surface
    d. Jumping on a trampoline

54. Which of the following statements is true about recovery time and training frequency for endurance clients?
    a. Clients training at a low intensity need the same number of training sessions but more recovery time than those training at a high intensity.
    b. Clients training at a high intensity need the same number of training sessions but more recovery time than those training at a low intensity.
    c. Both clients participating in high-intensity training and those doing low-intensity training need the same amount of recovery time.
    d. Clients who are doing high-intensity training sessions should get more time to recover and should train less frequently than low-intensity clients.

55. Interval training for aerobic clients and anaerobic clients is similar in which way?
    a. Intervals last the same amount of time for aerobic and anaerobic clients.
    b. Rest periods last the same amount of time for aerobic and anaerobic clients.
    c. Both types of clients are training at higher levels of intensity compared with their VO_2 max.
    d. Both types of clients use a 2:1 work-to-rest ratio.

56. Which of the following is not a benefit of free weights over resistance machines?
    a. They may be completed without a spotter.
    b. They can improve core stability.
    c. They can provide a more sports-specific strength training method.
    d. Each exercise can be performed in a variety of ways, rather than strictly dictated in one certain way.

57. For most strength exercises, which of the following breathing patterns is optimal?
    a. Inhale through the mouth during the concentric phase and exhale through the nose during the eccentric phase
    b. Exhale through the mouth during the concentric phase and inhale through the nose during the eccentric phase
    c. Inhale through the nose during the concentric phase and exhale through the mouth during the eccentric phase
    d. Exhale through the nose in the concentric phase and inhale through the mouth during the eccentric phase

58. Which of the following is NOT an adaptation to chronic cardiovascular conditioning?
    a. Increased heart chamber size
    b. Increased stroke volume
    c. Increased cardiac output
    d. Increased submaximal heart rate

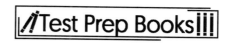

59. Golgi tendon organs are stimulated in PNF stretching and cause relaxation of which of the following?
   a. The antagonist muscle by its own contraction
   b. The stretched muscle by its own contraction
   c. The antagonist muscle by contracting the stretched muscle
   d. The stretched muscle by contracting the antagonist muscle

60. Spotters should be used for all EXCEPT which of the following exercises?
   a. Dumbbell chest press
   b. Incline barbell bench press
   c. Front squat
   d. Power jerk

61. Benefits of the Valsalva maneuver include all EXCEPT which of the following?
   a. Increases blood pressure
   b. Increases torso rigidity
   c. Decreases compressive forces on the intervertebral disks
   d. Supports the normal lordotic lumbar spine

62. During a heavy front-loaded squat, there should be how many spotter(s) who should be positioned in what location?
   a. 1, in the middle of the bar in front of the lifter
   b. 1, in the middle of the bar behind the lifter
   c. 2, on either end of the bar
   d. 2, one in front of and one behind the lifter

63. The number of required spotters is dependent on all EXCEPT which of the following?
   a. The load being lifted
   b. The number of strength coaches available
   c. The experience and skill of the client and spotters
   d. The physical strength of the spotters

64. When spotting over-the-face barbell exercises, the spotter should use what type of grip on the bar?
   a. Hook grip
   b. Pronated grip
   c. Alternated grip
   d. Supinated grip

65. Correct spotting position includes all BUT which of the following?
   a. Knees locked
   b. Feet flat on the floor
   c. Hands up in ready position
   d. Erect, neutral spine

66. Negative resistance training is best described as which of the following?
   a. Reducing training volume prior to competition to taper and improve performance
   b. A detraining effect that occurs when clients fail to train with high enough frequency
   c. Lifting heavier weights on the lowering, eccentric portion and getting assistance during the lifting, concentric phase
   d. Lifting heavier weights on the lifting, concentric portion and getting assistance during the lowering, eccentric phase

67. Benefits of bodyweight exercises include all BUT which of the following?
    a. They increase relative strength
    b. They increase absolute strength
    c. They can be performed on the field or away from the gym
    d. Clients can often complete many repetitions, improving muscular endurance

Answer Key and Explanations

1. C: Specificity in exercise training program refers to focusing exercises on improving the strength and power of muscle groups and movements unique to a specific sport or client's goals. For example, a competitive 50 m butterfly swimmer would heavily train the upper back and shoulders, isolating the rhomboids, deltoids, latissimus dorsi, levator scapulae, and multifidus.

2. B: As a client's fitness level improves, trainers employ program progression techniques, which keep the client adequately challenged so that improvement occurs. Trainers must reassess clients at regular intervals so that they can evaluate and modify the stimulus given in the training program. Modifications to the frequency, intensity, duration, and mode of exercise must occur consistently in order to avoid plateaus in training and ensure that the client remains challenged, and continues to improve in all areas of physical fitness.

3. B: Before engaging in an exercise-training program and in order to design and implement an effective and safe program, trainers must be familiar with the client's medical history. A trainer can best determine what exercises will be of maximum benefit and minimal risk of aggravating previous or current conditions by knowing all previous and current illnesses and injuries that the client has experienced.

4. D: Interval training involves workloads completed at a high level of exertion for brief periods interspersed with intermittent periods of rest, changing the speed and intensity of the workout. By challenging the cardiovascular and muscular systems to their maximum potential, providing only short rest periods, and then returning to high intensity efforts, interval training conditions the cardiovascular system, increases endurance, and maximizes metabolic functioning for improved weight loss.

5. D: Continuous training involves maintaining a steady speed and intensity of cardiovascular exercise. This type of training improves muscular endurance and metabolic functioning because the cardiovascular system is challenged for an extended period of time at a continuous effort.

6. C: Circuit training implements periods of cardiovascular exercise with intermittent strength training exercises. By challenging the cardiovascular system and muscular strength, circuit training also improves overall cardiovascular and muscular endurance, metabolic pathways, and muscular strength.

7. D: A Client's ADLs, or activities of daily living, should be considered when designing an effective and individualized exercise training program. If a client sits or stands for extended periods of time, performs repetitive motions throughout the day, uses upper or lower body muscle groups more than others, or has difficulty with movements in the early or late hours of the day, trainers may need to design specific exercises tailored to improve the client's quality of life. Such exercises may focus on cardiorespiratory fitness, strength, and/or flexibility.

8. B: For clients desiring weight loss, cardiovascular activity performed five to seven days per week is essential. Resistance training and flexibility exercises should also be components of the overall program along with a reduced-calorie diet.

9. A: Clients with goals of improving athletic performance require an exercise-training program that implements the principles of specificity and program progression. It should focus on the incorporation of exercises specific to the physical requirements of the intended sport.

10. C: Advanced resistance training methods can be useful for clients who have progressed through an exercise-training program and are ready for an additional challenge. Such advanced methods, such as kettlebells and supersets, improve fitness level and can help a client achieve his or her fitness goals, while providing variety and preventing boredom and plateaus.

11. B: Plyometric training requires the client to perform fast repetitions of speed- and power-focused exercises often with jumping and explosive movements such as box jumps and bounding drills.

12. D: Pyramid training involves high repetitions of exercises using a low weight, then progresses to fewer repetitions with a higher weight. These exercises can be performed in a variety of positions and can focus on a specific muscle group or all the major muscle groups.

13. A: Trainers should try to implement exercises to improve the client's efficiency and proper form. These supporting exercises should focus on the six motor skills related to physical fitness: agility, balance, coordination, reaction time, speed, and power.

14. B: The bench press is an example of a chest exercise. Back and chest muscles such as the pectoralis major and minor are targeted with exercises such as the bench press, dips, pull-ups, push-ups, and lat pull-downs.

15. C: The plank exercise is an example of an abdominal and core exercise. Abdominal muscles respond to core-focused exercises such as crunches, leg raises, and plank exercises. While planks can improve the strength and endurance of all major muscle groups used in maintaining proper posture during the plank, the core is mainly targeted in this isometric hold.

16. C: Pregnant women should consider modifying exercise after the first trimester. Pregnant clients with no contraindications are encouraged to continue to moderately exercise on a daily basis if they have done so before their pregnancy. Each trimester should be considered in order to make proper adjustments, such as discouraging supine exercises after the first trimester.

17. C: Range of motion exercises should be included in all training programs. Flexibility enables the body to perform movements in their full range of motion. Muscular strength and endurance play an integral role in optimal physical fitness by supporting the bone structure of the skeletal system and allowing for voluntary movements. Strength training helps maintain crucial muscle mass that can deteriorate with age and sedentary lifestyles.

18. A: Cardiovascular endurance refers to the ability of the cardiovascular system to efficiently pump blood throughout the body, delivering blood and essential oxygen to the muscles, tissues, and organs. Regular cardiovascular exercises such as swimming, running, and cycling strengthen this system and improves the functioning of all components (i.e. heart, blood vessels, arteries, etc.).

19. A: Strength training exercises improve muscular strength and endurance, and can be performed with body weight alone or a variety of external resistance modalities. Muscular strength and endurance play an integral part in physical fitness by supporting the skeletal system and allowing for voluntary movements; exercise programs can greatly improve the strength and endurance of muscles, helping to maintain crucial muscle mass that can deteriorate with age and inactivity.

20. D: Healthy populations such as adults, seniors, children, adolescents, and pregnant women should incorporate cardiovascular, resistance training, and flexibility in their programs. This balanced approach to fitness ensures the entire body is addressed and no imbalances are created.

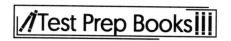

21. D: Clients with chronic conditions should incorporate low- to moderate-impact activities in their exercise program. Clients with a chronic disease will require medical clearance to engage in exercise, to ensure the safety and efficacy of the prescribed program.

22. A: Clients with arthritis and osteoporosis should engage in low-impact cardiovascular exercise for twenty to sixty minutes three to five days per week, gradually increasing the intensity and duration as the client's fitness and ability improve. Adequate rest should be taken if the client experiences any pain or discomfort before engaging in exercise again.

23. D: Obese clients should perform cardiovascular exercise five to seven days per week. The exercise should be performed at a moderate intensity for forty-five to sixty minutes. These exercises should be low-impact, such as swimming or walking, and should gradually include a wider variety of activities as the client's fitness improves. Risk of injury is greater in those with excessive body weight.

24. B: Warm-up, training, cool-down, stretching. A brief warm-up period of five to ten minutes allows a client to increase their cardiovascular activity and engage their muscles, helping to safely perform more rigorous activities efficiently during the workout. The main training stimulus comprises the bulk of the workout and follows the workout. It should include a variety of five to ten exercises involving the cardiovascular and musculoskeletal systems. Following the training stimulus stage, a cool-down at low-intensity permits the heart rate to return to normal, the metabolic byproducts of anaerobic respiration get shuttled to the liver, and the venous blood in the extremities returns to systemic circulation. Stretching the major muscle groups, as well as any specific muscles targeted in the workout, should end the training session, preventing lactic-acid buildup and discomfort.

25. A: By monitoring a client's heart rate, the trainer can determine whether an exercise's intensity, load, or duration should be modified. Asking the client to report their rate of perceived exertion (RPE) on a scale of six to twenty can also be useful in determining if modifications are necessary. Percentage of maximum oxygen consumption (also referred to as "VO_2 max") serves as a gauge of intensity by quantitative data that can be compared to previous and future measurements in an effort to record progress. Metabolic Equivalents (METs) help measure the activity energy expenditure compared to that of rest, providing another quantitative measure of exertion.

26. A: The arms and shoulder muscle include the biceps, triceps, deltoids, and trapezius. The hamstrings are in the posterior thigh.

27. D: The leg muscles include the quadriceps, hamstrings, and calf muscles. Deltoids are shoulder muscles.

28. A: The chest and back muscles include the deltoids, trapezius, pectoralis major and minor, latissimus dorsi, and rhomboids. The hamstrings are posterior thigh muscles.

29. D: The Borg RPE Scale determines a client's exertion on a scale of six to twenty. This can be useful in determining if modifications are required.

30. C: Age and pulse rate. When determining the appropriate exercise intensity, trainers can use the Karvonen Method and simply multiply the previously determined HRR by the percentage determined appropriate for training and then add the resting pulse. For example, a forty-year-old client needs to be trained at 80% of her HRR, her resting pulse is 70: 180 (her age-adjusted maximum heart rate); 180-70 (resting pulse) = 110; 110 x .80 = 88 + 70 (resting pulse rate) = 158 bpm.

31. C: Periodization refers to the intensity levels of exercises per period or cycle of training. Periodized training programs consist of certain periods designated for specific skills, strengths, or movements and then modified to address new skills or a different focus in the next period. For example, the first period of an athlete's periodized program might focus on strength and endurance, the second on agility and speed, the third on mastering fine motor skills and coordination, and the last might address skills unique to the client's specific sport. While these periodized portions of the program should have specific areas of focus, a trainer should ensure that the client continues to perform and progress in the exercises focused on cardiovascular fitness, strength training, and flexibility simultaneously.

32. A: Clients can generally benefit from a basic training load of 55% to 85% of their one-repetition maximum. Modifications should be made to limit the risk of injury. In order to design an effective exercise-training program, a trainer must be able to determine the appropriate repetitions, sets, loads, and rest periods for exercises based on the client's skills, abilities, restrictions, and goals.

33. B: For improving endurance, the general recommendation is to perform two to three sets of fifteen repetitions or more within the weight load range of 55% to 65% of the client's 1 repetition maximum. All sets should be performed with a rest interval of two to four minutes between sets.

34. A: For muscle hypertrophy, three to six sets of six to twelve repetitions at 75% of the 1 repetition maximum is recommended. For increases in strength, two to six sets of fewer than six repetitions performed at 75% to 85% of the 1 repetition maximum is effective. Power training entails three to five sets of one to two repetitions performed at 90% to 100% of 1 repetition maximum. All sets should be performed with a resting period of two to four minutes between, with exception of power-related sets, which require one minute of rest between.

35. B: Hygiene is not included in the components of physical fitness. Physical fitness is composed of a number of aspects of health that synergistically support the body in functioning at its best. Cardiovascular endurance, muscle strength, flexibility, and body composition all play a part in contributing to the body's ability to perform.

36. C: When developing the ideal exercise-training program for a client who has sports-specific goals, the components of the training regimen should focus on improving the endurance, strength, power, and flexibility of the client in order to maximize the body's ability in performing physical movements most commonly executed in their specific sport.

37. A: Anaerobic exercises include explosive exercises performed for only short durations and require little-to-no oxygen delivery to the muscles throughout the performance. Aerobic exercises require oxygen in order to perform for extended periods of time such as running, swimming, and bicycling.

38. B: Aerobic exercises, such as running, swimming, and endurance cycling, require oxygen in order to perform for extended periods of time. Anaerobic exercises include explosive exercises performed for only short durations and require little-to-no oxygen delivery to the muscles throughout the performance.

39. B: If a client reports new-onset discomfort in the chest and arms, the appropriate action of the trainer would be to seek medical assistance. While this symptom can be considered a fairly normal physical response to vigorous exercise, trainers are responsible for recognizing when a client's symptoms may indicate a serious medical complication. When in doubt, trainers should err on the side of caution and refer the client to a physician for approval to continue with the exercise program. This prioritizes the client's health and minimizes the risk of liability for the trainer.

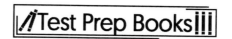

40. A: Training clients at higher altitudes can result in dehydration. Additionally, clients may experience limited respiratory capabilities and compromised equilibrium (balance). Paying close attention to the client's level of perceived exertion, proper form, and hydration, the trainer can implement breaks as needed, instruct the client to hydrate more frequently, and minimize risks associated with exercise at altitude.

41. B: Teachability is not included in the four components of the FITT principle. The four components of the FITT principle are: Frequency, Intensity, Time, and Type. The FITT principle can guide trainers in the design, implementation, and modification of a client's exercise training program to ensure that the client remains challenged, progresses toward their fitness and health goals, minimizes the risk of injury or illness, and avoid plateaus in fitness level.

42. D: Core exercises can improve a client's strength across his or her whole body in addition to specific muscle groups. However, sleep deprivation, lack of nutrition, and overtraining can all reduce a client's ability to increase training load. Rest is an important part of strength training and can help a client prevent overtraining. Proper nutrition is essential for fueling the workout and providing the building blocks for developing more muscle mass.

43. B: The heart-rate reserve increases and the resting heart rate decreases. Heart-rate reserve is defined as the difference between the maximal heart rate and the resting heart rate. Even though heart rate initially increases during exercise, resting heart rate decreases as a person adapts to aerobic activity. As resting heart rate decreases, the heart rate reserve will increase because the difference between maximal and resting heart rate will increase.

44. C: Longer resting periods improve cardiovascular conditioning. When a client needs to improve cardiovascular conditioning, he or she may decrease resting time to bolster aerobic endurance.

45. A: Training for muscular hypertrophy requires six to twelve repetitions. Completing more than twelve repetitions improves muscle endurance, while doing fewer than six repetitions improves strength as long as the resistance lifted poses the appropriate challenge at the given repetition level. Using three different exercises per muscle group can significantly increase muscle growth.

46. B: Muscle balance is crucial for any strength-training program because a lack of balance causes the body to have abnormal movement patterns and increases the risk of injury. Creating muscle balance means to improve strength ratios between opposing muscle groups. An example of muscle balance is a 3:4 strength ratio between hamstrings and quadriceps.

47. D: Multi-joint exercises stimulate muscles the most and allow for the greatest amount of loading during resistance training. Primary exercises are core exercises that are sport-specific and involve large muscle groups and multiple joints. Structural exercises are core exercises that load the spine. Assistance exercises engage small muscle groups and single joints.

48. C: Circuit training improves mental focus and requires a client to do a variety of exercises (from most intense to least intense) with little rest in between sets. This training program improves cardiorespiratory function and has a high metabolic cost, which leads to increased body-fat loss.

49. A: Exercises should be ordered from most to least technical, with power movements first, core exercises second, and single-joint exercises last. Olympic lifts are power movements and require extensive technique, whereas biceps curls require little technique and involve a single joint.

50. C: Performing an exercise for at least twelve repetitions will improve muscular endurance, whereas six to twelve repetitions will enhance muscular hypertrophy and fewer than six repetitions will improve muscular strength.

51. A: Training intensity must be decreased to improve speed. Increasing training volume and changing the duration of rest periods between sets will also promote physical adaptations in the client.

52. B: The unloading/deloading week uses lower training volumes and decreases intensity so that the client can recover and be prepared for future training sessions. This training week allows the client to continue improving neural patterns and promotes supercompensation.

53. D: Doing exercises on an unstable or uneven surface (e.g., doing bodyweight squats or push-ups on a BOSU) helps to improve neuromuscular control by stimulating and challenging the nervous system in new ways, which necessitates adaptation.

54. D: The greater the intensity of training, the more recovery time the client needs before the next training session. Therefore, clients training at high intensity should have fewer training sessions per week tha clients training low intensities.

55. C: Interval training involves working at higher levels of intensity compared with one's VO_2 max. Interval lengths and rest periods are very different. Aerobic clients use a 1:1 work/rest ratio during interval training.

56. A: Exercises with free weights should use a minimum of one or two spotters when a client moves the bar over the head or face, has it on the front of the shoulders, or has it on the back during the execution. Resistance machines frequently do not need a spotter because they have safety features designed into them, but for certain maximal lifts, a spotter is recommended. Free weight training can improve core stability and can provide a more sports-specific strength training method. Each exercise can be performed in a variety of ways, rather than strictly dictated in one specific way.

57. B: For most strength exercises, the client should exhale through the mouth during the concentric phase through the sticking point and then inhale through the nose during the eccentric phase. Breathing should be slow and controlled.

58. D: Increased submaximal heart rate is not a chronic adaptation to cardiovascular exercise. In fact, heart rate decreases at a given submaximal workload due to improvements in cardiorespiratory economy. Heart chamber size increases, as does preload (the amount of blood that fills a chamber before it contracts to eject it), resulting in a higher stroke volume per heartbeat. This means that more blood, oxygen, and nutrients get moved per pump of the heart. Blood volume and hemoglobin content of the blood also increase.

59. B: Golgi tendon organs are stimulated in PNF stretching and cause relaxation of the stretched muscle by its own contraction.

60. D: Spotters are not used in power exercises such as the power jerk. With the exception of power exercises, free weight exercises should use a minimum of one or two spotters when a client moves the bar over the head or face, has it on the front of the shoulders, or on the back during the execution. During power exercises, client should be instructed to push the bar away or drop it when the bar is in front, and release it or jump forward when the bar is missed behind the head; a spotter should not be used.

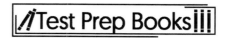

61. A: The Valsalva maneuver can be used in certain core exercises with care as a way to increase torso rigidity to aid in support of the vertebral column, which lessens compressive forces on the intervertebral discs and supports the normal and neutral lordotic lumbar spine. Blood pressure can increase with the Valsalva maneuver, but this is not a benefit, and in fact, can cause undesirable dizziness and disorientation.

62. C: During a heavy front-loaded squat, there should be 2 spotters – one positioned on either end of the bar – to help balance it and to remain in constant communication with each other and the lifter.

63. B: The required number of spotters is determined by the load being lifted, the experience and skill of the client and spotters, and the physical strength of the spotters. The spotters must be strong enough to handle the load that the client is lifting with little notice and sometimes in less than ideal angles and positions, so it is crucial that spotters are honest with themselves and the lifter about their abilities. It is safer to err on the side of caution and use multiple spotters when necessary, as long as they can be accommodated spatially around the lift without being overly cumbersome.

64. C: When spotting over-the-face barbell exercises, the spotter should use the alternated grip pattern, usually narrower than the client's grip. In this position, one hand is supinated and one is pronated.

65. A: Spotters should use a solid, wide base of support and a neutral spine position. Spotters should use an athletic stance, with feet slightly wider than hip width apart, knees flexed, arms and hands up and in the ready position and as close to the bar and client without touching them as possible. Bodyweight should be equally and soundly distributed on both feet, which should be firmly planted on the ground. Knees should not be locked but should maintain a degree of flexion, ready to support the weight and go into a squat if necessary to accept the weight of the bar. Locking the knees can be dangerous, since it places excessive stress on the knee ligaments and cartilage as well as the lower leg muscles and bones and the low back.

66. C: Negative resistance training is best described as lifting heavier weights on the lowering, eccentric portion and getting assistance from spotters during the lifting, concentric phase. It is a specific resistance training protocol based on the concept that most clients can handle heavier loads on the eccentric portions of exercises, but are not able to lift the load concentrically, so they need assistance. However, if they are only to use the load they can handle concentrically, they are never fully challenging the stronger eccentrically working muscles, so negative resistance training addresses this discrepancy. It is an advanced lifting technique.

67. B: Bodyweight training such as pull-ups, push-ups, chin-ups, squat thrusts, lunges, yoga, jumping jacks, and planks provide resistance in the form of bodyweight, so it improves relative strength and core strength, is low-cost, and improves body control. Because there are not external weights used, it does not improve absolute strength.

Exercise Leadership & Client Education

Creating a Positive Exercise Experience to Optimize Adherence

Keeping the client motivated in his or her exercise program and applying behavioral change are keys to adherence. Trainers can foster a positive, supportive environment by using a variety of verbal and nonverbal communication techniques. Use of S.M.A.R.T. (Specific, Measurable, Attainable, Realistic, and Timely) goals and tapping into sources of intrinsic and extrinsic motivational aids, helping ensure the client has a dependable support system, giving frequent reinforcement and feedback, and identifying and tackling barriers to adherence can bolster client success.

Learning Styles

There are different learning styles that can vary with each client. The trainer should be aware of these learning styles because a client will greatly benefit from instructions during sessions that are tailored to his or her specific learning style. Auditory learners learn through hearing, so the trainer can explain exercises and give verbal cues about form. Visual learners learn through seeing, so the trainer can demonstrate and exercise for the client to observe and give printed illustrations of exercises for the client to take home and review. Kinesthetic learners learn through movement, involvement, and experience. The trainer can demonstrate and then have the client try an unweighted trial of the exercise or a partial range of motion to demonstrate understanding before trying the full resistance or movement.

Health Behavior Change Models to Support Exercise Adherence

An understanding of behavioral change models will assist personal trainers in reinforcing positive behaviors and help clients avoid sabotaging progress toward behavioral goals. While there are many health behavioral change models, several common ones (as discussed before) and the ways in which they can be used to support exercise adherence are as follows:

Health Belief Model: The perceived seriousness of a potential health problem is the main predictor of behavioral change, aided by discussions of the physical and psychological benefits of exercise and the consequences of inactivity.

Theory of Planned Behavior: The client's level of motivation for behavioral change is shaped by his or her attitudes, subjective norms, and perceived control. The intention to engage in a behavior will ultimately result in that behavior. Plans such as carrying extra exercise clothes and shoes in the car to be ready when opportunity strikes, formally scheduling workouts into a calendar, and planning for high-risk relapse situations (like packing exercise DVDs and a resistance band for work travel) use this model to encourage adherence.

Social Cognitive Theory: Behavioral change is influenced by the triad of interactions of the environment, personal factors, and behavior itself. It relies heavily on the idea of self-efficacy. Self-regulatory strategies such as self-monitoring physical activity, setting personal goals and rewards, planning activity in advance, and having reasonable expectations are methods using this theory to improve adherence.

Socio-Ecological Model: Addresses relationships. Behaviors, such as a client's motivation to exercise, are shaped by interpersonal relations, the surrounding environment, community, policy, and law. To

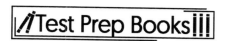

improve adherence, make sure the client has a good social support system, perhaps has an exercise buddy, goes to a gym in a convenient location to work or home, or perhaps joins a local sports league.

Barriers to Exercise Adherence and Compliance

Barriers to exercise adherence and compliance can be personal (fear, embarrassment, injury), behavioral (lack of motivation, unhealthy habits in times of stress, time management), environmental (no safe parks near client's home, inconvenient gyms), social (lack of support or someone sabotaging progress), and programmatic (lack of knowledge, too intense of a previous plan that caused injury or failure). Trainers should help clients identify the barriers in their own lives and brainstorm solutions such as designing home exercise programs or "on-the-road" workouts for traveling, eliciting social support, offering helpful rewards and incentives, and educating clients on alternative workout locations or dietary substitutions. The solutions should be mutually evaluated, since some will be more realistic than others. The trainer should aid the client in developing a plan for implementing solutions to the identified barriers. After that step, the plan may need to be fine-tuned.

Relapses

Some breaks in an exercise routine are inevitable, such as with injury, illness, travel, or holidays, but it may be possible to circumnavigate others, such as inclement weather or a busier work schedule. Interruptive events can cause relapse, but if psychological, behavioral, or physical strategies are employed in advance to ensure such breaks are only temporary and do not become full-blown lapses, the client can continue training and resume a path toward success of his or her fitness goals.

Trainers should emphasize that these breaks or relapses are not failures as long as the routine is picked up again as soon as possible. If not, arrangements and modifications to the plan can be made to accommodate some of these challenges, enabling the client to stay focused and remain motivated toward achieving his or her goals. Trainers should remind clients of the physical and psychological benefits of exercise, possibly implement reward strategies, and ensure that the client has the social support to get back on the program. Sometimes perceived failure or lack of progress can cause a client to relapse into a sedentary lifestyle. If so, it might be necessary to re-evaluate the goals and shift focus to something more rewarding or tangible in the short-term. This will instill a feeling of success before moving back toward tackling a particularly challenging goal.

Techniques to Facilitate Motivation

Trainers can employ a variety of techniques to facilitate client motivation, depending on the client's personality and challenges as well as his or her stage of readiness (transtheoretical model). In earlier stages, rewards may need to be more tangible and frequent. As the client moves more from the preparation and action stage to the maintenance stage, the focus can shift to more of the rewarding aspects of exercises such as enjoyment, improvements in health, and a break from the workday. Some motivational techniques include the following:

- In early stages of a program: use of a points system, competitions, recognitions (Athlete of the Month bulletin board), trophies

- Personal contracts

- Varied routines to prevent boredom and burnout or exercise challenges

- Reminders of the benefits of exercise or the negatives of inactivity

- Well-rounded S.M.A.R.T goals that are both long-term and short-term, addressing all five areas of health-related fitness

- Social support such as group classes, buddy systems, periodic telephone calls or emails, support from family and friends

- External rewards such as new exercise clothes, playlists, spa treatments if certain weekly physical activity recommendations are met

- Reduced fees or free sessions based on adherence

Extrinsic and Intrinsic Reinforcement Strategies

Rewards and reinforcements may help in motivating clients to make and keep positive behavioral changes. Extrinsic rewards are factors outside of the exercise itself that help to support the desire to be physically active, and may be especially important in the earlier stages of programs when the exercise itself is more painful due to discomfort and lower fitness levels. Extrinsic rewards include things like a free t-shirt or iTunes gift card for workout music, which can be given after completing a certain number of sessions. It is important that such rewards are not counterproductive to accomplishing health goals — for example, high-calorie milkshakes or candy bars. Intrinsic rewards are ones the client feels directly from the exercise itself, such as improved self-esteem or fitting into their favorite jeans. These rewards remain important long after goal achievement. Intrinsically motivated clients or those with self-determination enjoy the process of the exercise itself and therefore may maintain their health behaviors more easily than externally motivated clients who exercise for the sake of achieving some sort of reward. As the client's fitness level improves, it is likely that extrinsic rewards may become less important.

Strategies to Increase Non-Structured Physical Activity

Trainers can encourage clients to add unstructured physical activity throughout the day by making "healthy swaps," which means replacing a sedentary behavior with a healthy, active one. Some suggestions include:

- Wearing a pedometer or using a phone app to track activity with the goal of increasing steps per day
- Engaging in active play with children or grandchildren
- Keeping an extra pair of workout clothes and sneakers in the car for spontaneous opportunities to be active
- Walking a dog, walking at lunch, getting up to walk around a few minutes every hour
- Performing yard work such as gardening, raking, shoveling, pruning, cleaning gutters
- Performing housework such as vacuuming, mopping, dusting, rearranging furniture
- Walking or biking to the corner store for milk or small groceries instead of driving
- Walking to local establishments for food instead of ordering delivery
- Walking or biking to work if the commute is reasonably short
- If taking public transportation, getting off a few stops early to a destination to walk the remainder
- Refraining from emailing or calling coworkers and walking to their desk instead
- Taking stairs instead of elevators
- Parking farther away from the entrance at stores or work

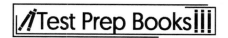

Health Coaching Principles

Research has found that motivational interviewing is a successful tool for improving readiness for changing health behaviors such as engaging in or increasing exercise. This technique involves acknowledging and slowly working through a client's challenges concerning regular activity, stressing the fact that it is his or her choice to be active while also encouraging the change. Motivational interviewing requires clients to reflect on what may happen if they do not change their current habits and weighs the pros and cons of activity and inactivity. Personal trainers can also use the Five A's Model when counseling clients to create a physical activity plan:

- Address why the client is there. What is the agenda?
- Assess current health and activity and readiness for change
- Advise clients of the benefits of activity and consequences of inactivity
- Assist clients in creating a plan for exercise and conquering barriers
- Arrange for follow-up after plan implementation

Leadership Techniques and Educating Clients

One of the primary functions of a personal trainer is to educate clients by using research-based health and fitness information. As a client's knowledge base grows, increases are generally seen in enjoyment, adherence, awareness, and application of such health and fitness advice to the exercise program and a healthy lifestyle. Trainers should strive to stay current with research and continuing education and embody the mindset that educating clients is an ongoing process and should not be a one-time event.

Active Listening Techniques

Active listening is a process of trying to understand the underlying meaning in a client's words, which builds empathy and trust as well as greater client satisfaction and compliance. Asking open-ended questions and repeating or rephrasing what a client said in a reflective or clarifying manner is a form of active listening that builds a positive, trusting relationship. The client may indicate he or she would like to "lose a few pounds," and, in response, the trainer could ask, "Okay, so just to make sure we are in the same page, it sounds like you are hoping to lose a little weight?" The trainer should encourage the client with verbal and nonverbal cues, eye contact and undivided attention, look engaged and non-judgmental, and not rush the client.

Types of Feedback to Optimize Training

Written reports and verbal feedback are important in the process of goal achievement. They also correct and teach proper form. They should be given at frequent intervals so the client can have knowledge of his or her progress and stay motivated toward the goals. Feedback should be timely while the movement or assessment is fresh in the client's mind. Feedback should always be given in positive language and never come across as threatening.

The following are common forms of feedback and how they might be used in sessions:

Evaluative feedback: guides the client to make improvements on incorrect movements or form and understands what parts he or she is mastering. Example: "Your back is perfectly straight now, but let's see if you can bring your hands closer to shoulder-width apart."

Supportive feedback: often given during particularly difficult parts of a workout as a means of encouraging the client. Example: "I know it's challenging, but if you can push through three more reps, you will break your record!"

Descriptive feedback: given at the completion of a movement or workout in a clean, concise fashion that provides a summary of what was seen and what can be improved or changed. After completing biceps curls, the trainer may remark, "It's exciting to see you working hard on these curls. I notice as you get tired, there's a tendency to swing the weights forward and use momentum. Let's see if we can use a little bit of a lighter weight next set and try to focus on isolating your biceps to bring the weight up."

Corrective feedback: should be given immediately, especially if something is unsafe. Example: "It seems like you are yanking up on your neck during these crunches, but your hands should just be supporting your head, not pulling it up."

Communication Modes

Phone calls, emails, text messages, newsletters, and websites are all useful tools that facilitate frequent conversations with clients, although each client may have his or her communication mode preferences. The trainer can likely find ways to incorporate a variety of these methods. Electronic or digital means such as text and email are convenient and fast. They may be used in ways such as to remind clients of upcoming sessions, notify clients to bring something to a session, such as an extra water bottle, or as a way to offer friendly and quick praise after a great session. Phone calls may work better for longer discussions, perhaps when a client is sick and the trainer is giving return-to-activity advice, or if the client is not easily reachable by digital means. Confidentiality principles should always be practiced. Trainers should not send sensitive or personal messages through any method that may breach this need. Newsletters and websites are geared more toward a wider audience, rather than the individual client, although clients may use these resources to learn more about nutrition, exercises, or other informative articles the trainer prepares. These communication channels can also be used as marketing tools for the trainer to recruit new clients. Plus, the trainer can employ metrics to analyze the reach and return-on-investment for such sources.

Influence of Lifestyle Factors on Lipid and Lipoprotein Profiles

Genetics can predispose a client to hypercholesterolemia and high blood lipid levels, although epigenetics (how the genes are turned on and off and are expressed) can be altered by lifestyle, nutrition, and physical activity. As clients move from a sedentary lifestyle and poor dietary choices to a more active, healthy lifestyle and improved nutrition intake, lipid profiles will improve. It is not uncommon for clients who take lipid-lowering medications to enjoy the benefits of no longer needing such medications as a result of increased activity from an exercise program as well as dietary improvements.

Carbohydrates, Fats, and Proteins as Fuels for Exercise

Carbohydrates and fats are the primary macronutrients used to fuel exercise. The breakdown of these substrates provides adenosine triphosphate (ATP) for the body to do work. Carbohydrates are the body's preferred energy source for most aerobic and anaerobic exercise, both during resistance and cardiovascular exercise. At very low levels of exertion, such as during walking, yoga, and gentle cycling, fats provide a greater proportion of the energy requirements. The body can only store a limited amount of carbohydrates in the form of muscle and liver glycogen (generally about 2000 kcal worth, depending

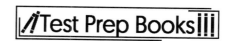

on training status and body size), so as these stores deplete, reliance on fat and protein for energy increase. By ingesting some carbohydrates during extended endurance exercise, such as in marathon training or on long bike rides, the body can continue to have an ample supply of carbohydrates to prevent "hitting the wall" experiences that occur as energy levels drop when the body runs out of glycogen to feed into the Krebs Cycle and starts needing to use fat and protein more. These two substrates are slower burning fuels, so the intensity level permitted while burning these fuels is lower, resulting in decreased performance and speed.

Dietary and Body Fat Terms

The following terms are important for trainers to be knowledgeable about effective communication as allied health professionals. It should be noted that Anorexia and Bulimia Nervosa are serious eating disorders that can be fatal and necessitate care from medical and mental health professionals. Here are some common terms related to body fat:

Body Composition: the relative proportion of fat mass and fat-free mass of the body. Typically, women have a higher percentage of body fat than men.

Body Mass Index (BMI): a relation or measure of body weight (in kilograms) divided by height (in meters squared). It is used to classify individuals into underweight, normal weight, overweight, and obese groups with varying corresponding disease risk.

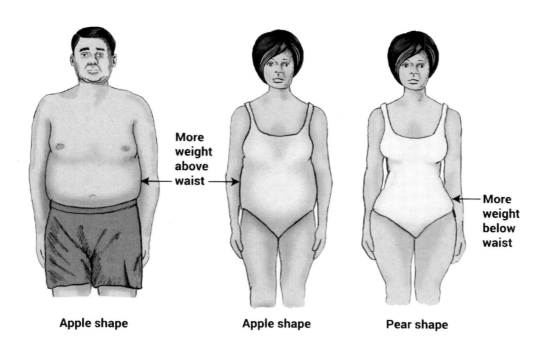

Lean Body Mass: the fat-free mass of the body, including, but not limited to, bone, muscle, organs, blood, and tissue

Anorexia Nervosa: an eating or body image disorder consisting of starvation and inadequate nutritive intake; a component of a syndrome called female athlete triad (with amenorrhea and decreased bone density)

Bulimia Nervosa: an eating disorder characterized by binging and purging behavior (induced vomiting, or unnecessary use of laxatives)

Body Fat Distribution: the specific pattern or locations of adipose tissue on the body; typically because of hormonal profiles, women carry more fat on their hips and thighs (gynoid or pear-shaped) while men carry more abdominal fat (android or apple-shaped).

Relationship Between Body Composition and Health

Both excessive total fat (overweight and obesity) and abdominal (visceral) fat distribution negatively impact health and can increase risk of cardiovascular and metabolic diseases, musculoskeletal injuries, and certain cancers, therefore increasing the risk of morbidity and mortality. At a BMI of 30 kg/m^2 or greater, the mortality rate increases 50 to 100 percent. Male and female bodies have essential fat levels. These serve as the minimal body fat percentages needed to sustain life and support the organs, tissues, and systems of the body. Excessively low body fat and body water percentages, resulting from malnutrition or eating disorders, can also be dangerous. These types of severely restrictive behaviors can be seen in wrestlers, dancers, gymnasts, distance runners, and other athletes who trainers may work with.

The following are standards for body fat percentages and, above these levels, people are considered overweight and obese:

Men:

- Essential: 3 to 5 percent
- Athletic: 5 to 13 percent
- Recommended (less than 35 years old): 8 to 22 percent, obese: greater than 25 percent
- Recommended (35 or more years old): 10 to 25 percent, obese: greater than 28 percent

Women:

- Essential: 8 to 12 percent
- Athletic: 12 to 22 percent
- Recommended (less than 35 years old): 20 to 35 percent, obese: greater than 38 percent
- Recommended (35 or more years old): 23 to 38 percent, obese: greater than 40 percent

Modifying Body Composition via Diet, Exercise, and Behavior

Research has found that both restricted calorie diets and increased physical activity programs can result in a reduction in weight and body fat, and a combination of these programs may be the most successful approach. When interventions have a behavioral component — such as teaching goal-setting, self-efficacy, reducing barriers to a healthy lifestyle, and reliance on social support — weight loss results seem to be maintained for a longer time after program completion because the participant has the tools and strategies in place to persevere in his or her weight loss efforts, rather than reverting back to unhealthy habits. The exercise component may not only reduce body fat, but also preserve muscle mass, which keeps metabolic rate from dropping and improves overall body composition.

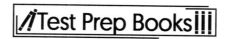

Hydration

Hydration is important before, during, and after exercise not only for performance, but also for optimal health. A loss of 3 to 5 percent body weight in water may be tolerated without a corresponding loss of maximal strength, but moderate or severe dehydration (loss of greater than 5 percent body weight) can lead to decreased endurance capacity, decreased heat tolerance, and increased injury risk. Sweat rate can be estimated by weighing the body before and after exercise and subtracting any fluid consumed during exercise. While it is ideal to match fluid intake to body weight in ounces lost, clients should drink a minimum of one pint for each pound of lost weight to mitigate the effects of more substantial dehydration. Water is usually sufficient, but for prolonged activities over an hour or in particularly hot climates, sports drinks with electrolytes are a more appropriate choice.

Dietary Guidelines

The USDA publishes Dietary Guidelines for Healthy Americans every several years, with changes as nutrition science advances. The Food Guide Pyramid has been replaced by ChooseMyPlate.gov and provides tips and guidelines for portion sizes and relative amounts in each food group to strive for, as well as recommended amounts of physical activity. The full report and printable resources that trainers can share with clients are available at: cnpp.usda.gov/2015-2020-dietary-guidelines-americans

Female Athlete Triad

Disordered eating leads to insufficient energy intake, causing amenorrhea (loss of menstrual cycle) and decreased bone density (osteopenia or osteoporosis), which are the three cornerstones of the female athlete triad. If trainers suspect any of these issues, they should refer the client to medical professionals. Calorie restriction from disordered eating leads to low energy levels and when body fat gets too low, estrogen levels drop, and a loss of menses (amenorrhea) occurs. The menstrual cycle and estrogen levels are important in supporting healthy bone mineral density by depositing calcium into the bony matrix. With prolonged amenorrhea, calcium is depleted from bones and they are susceptible to fractures. Overall health suffers and injury risk (ligament, tendon, and muscle injuries) increases when the female is in negative energy balance (expending more calories than ingesting). While the role of trainers is often to encourage exercise, this is an instance when exercise may need to be restricted.

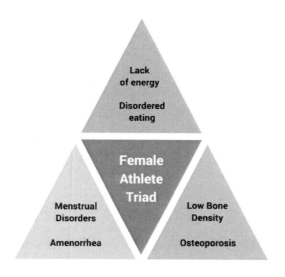

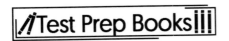

Inappropriate Weight Loss Methods

Unfortunately, fad diets are popularized in the media on a daily basis. The weight-loss industry is a multi-billion-dollar industry for a reason: people are desperate to lose weight and are often looking for a "quick, easy fix," which many of these diets and exercise gadgets promise. However, many of these fad diets are dangerous or not developed by consummate professionals with any scientific research to validate their safety or efficacy, eliminating entire food groups or claiming the diet to be some sort of health panacea. Other unhealthy methods promising rapid weight loss in popular culture include exercising in saunas or steam rooms to "sweat off pounds," starvation or liquid diets, cleanses, and mega dosing dietary supplements. These can cause dangerous dehydration, overdose on certain supplements, electrolyte imbalances that can cause arrhythmias, and loss of resting metabolic rate when the body senses starvation, making subsequent weight loss harder. Trainers should be aware that clients may inquire about such diets and fitness gadgets. When they do, trainers should remember that it may take patience as well as targeted and thorough education to convey the danger and ineffectiveness of such methods and provide the alternative realities for healthy weight loss.

Kilocalories in Carbohydrates, Fats, Proteins and Alcohol

The various macronutrients have different calories (kcal) per gram, which can be important to consider for dietary recommendations and when reading nutrition labels. Carbohydrates and proteins provide four calories per gram, alcohol has seven, and fats provide nine calories per gram.

Guidelines for Caloric Intake for Weight Loss or Weight Gain

The American Council on Exercise (ACE) recommends a daily calorie deficit of 500 to 1000 kcal for those looking to lose weight. This can be achieved through increased energy expenditure via activity and/or reduced caloric intake. Because each pound of fat has 3500 kcal, this should result in one to two pounds of weight per week. Faster rates are not recommended because they may result in loss of lean body mass and body water as well as fat mass. This can slow metabolism because muscle mass contributes to a higher metabolic rate than fat mass. A loss of one to two pounds per week preserves lean body mass and also improves adherence, since it typically is due to maintainable lifestyle changes rather than drastic starvation methods that are unhealthy and not sustainable, resulting in weight regain.

Calorie restricting diets should emphasize healthy, nutrient-rich foods such as vegetables, fruits, legumes, lean proteins, and healthy fats as well as ample water for hydration. It is not just calories—processed foods and empty calories such as chemically laden "diet foods" and sodas should be avoided, even if they appear to have lower calorie counts. Suggested rates of weight gain are similar and should also be achieved through healthy food choices, focusing on nutrient-dense foods such as nuts, seeds, vegetables, grains, fruits, and healthy fats. Calories expended during exercise need to be replaced. Clients may find that drinking calorie-rich beverages such as milk, almond milk, and pressed juices can be helpful.

Scientifically-Based Health Resources

There are a variety of scientifically-based journals that trainers can subscribe to in order to stay current in the health and fitness fields. These publications cover information, studies, and procedures, enabling the trainer to provide the best care and instruction for clients.

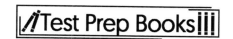

Community-Based Exercise Programs

The personal trainer should research and establish connections with local community-based exercise programs, since these can provide social support through recreational and structured activities to augment clients' physical activity outside of scheduled exercise sessions. Many communities have affordable walking or running clubs, intramural sports, recreation leagues, or bowling teams for a variety of ages and levels. Trainers should encourage clients to try a variety of programs and activities to find a personally enjoyable form of exercise. Some programs, such as strength training classes, may also have an interest or need for trainers.

Stress Management and Relaxation Techniques

Acute and chronic stress are inevitable. Trainers should have a list of referrals and develop relationships with local professionals to recommend to clients, such as licensed massage therapists, Reiki practitioners, acupuncturists, and mental health professionals. Trainers can also suggest apps, books, or guides for progressive relaxation, mindfulness meditation, or guided imagery. As allied health professionals and supporters of behavioral change, trainers should be prepared to be supportive, empathetic, and active listeners for clients who want to share about life stresses and vent during sessions. While trainers can help brainstorm and provide suggested solutions for clients to consider, it is important that trainers try to guide clients in a way that allows the client to take ownership in the problem-solving process in order to build self-efficacy.

Practice Questions

1. Which of the following is NOT a way to foster a positive exercise experience?
    a. Using S.M.A.R.T. goals
    b. Using infrequent reinforcement and feedback
    c. Identifying barriers to adherence and strategizing solutions
    d. Building a support

2. Which of the following includes all of the appropriate methods of communication with clients?
    a. Email, phone, text messaging, in person
    b. Phone, in person
    c. Email, in person, phone
    d. In person, text messaging, phone

3. Which would be best for a kinesthetic learner?
    a. Reading about proper squatting technique
    b. Trying to squat back into a chair before a full body squat
    c. Watching video tutorials of squatting form
    d. Listening to you explain the major form tips for a perfect squat

4. A visual learner would probably prefer which of the following?
    a. Reading about proper squatting technique
    b. Trying to squat back into a chair before a full body squat
    c. Watching video tutorials of squatting form
    d. Listening to you explain the major form tips for a perfect squat

5. Which is an example of active listening to a client who says, "I would like to lose a little weight and get in shape"?
    a. "Okay, good. Why don't you tell me what a typical day looks like for you?"
    b. "Okay, don't worry. That's certainly understandable."
    c. "Okay, so it sounds like you are interested in improving your fitness and losing a little weight. Can you tell me more about that?"
    d. "Okay. According to your BMI, I think we should aim for 40 pounds."

6. "I know it's challenging, but if you can push through three more reps, you will break your record!" is an example of what type of feedback?
    a. Evaluative
    b. Supportive
    c. Descriptive
    d. Corrective

7. "Your back is perfectly straight now, but let's see if you can bring your hands closer to shoulder-width apart." is an example of what type of feedback?
    a. Evaluative
    b. Supportive
    c. Descriptive
    d. Corrective

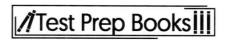

8. John is 5'10" and 210 pounds. According to the BMI, he would be categorized as which of the following?
    a. Underweight
    b. Normal weight
    c. Overweight
    d. Obese

9. "Feedback should be timely" is best described by which of the following statements?
    a. It should be given after every session
    b. It should be given after assessments only to explain results
    c. It should be given sporadically so it doesn't lose its meaning
    d. It should be given during or soon after a movement or assessment

10. Which of the following categories of barriers to a healthy lifestyle can trainers likely have the greatest impact on?
    a. Environmental
    b. Programmatic
    c. Social
    d. Personal

11. Ensuring the client has a good social support system, such as an exercise buddy, a gym in a convenient location to work or home, or a local sports league membership are methods to improve adherence based on which behavioral change model?
    a. Socio-Ecological Model
    b. Theory of Planned Behavior
    c. Social Cognitive Theory
    d. Health Belief Model

12. Which of the following is NOT a good way to prevent relapses in exercise behavior?
    a. Making goals easily achievable
    b. Assuring clients that short lapses are inevitable and not failures
    c. Ensuring a client's social support system is positive
    d. Making a list of possible causes of relapses and brainstorming solutions

13. Which of the following is NOT a reason that relapses in exercise behavior occur?
    a. Too much intrinsic motivation
    b. Lack of social support
    c. Illness or injury
    d. Perceived sense of failure

14. Tina is a new client who had a previously sedentary life. Which might be the best choice of a technique to facilitate motivation?
    a. Reducing session fees after she completes twenty sessions
    b. Reminding her of the benefits of exercise and the risks of inactivity
    c. Making S.M.A.R.T. fitness goals after assessment
    d. Establishing a points system to win prizes after completing sessions each week

15. Self-regulatory strategies such as self-monitoring physical activity and setting personal goals and rewards, planning activity in advance, and having reasonable expectations are methods to improve adherence based on which behavioral change model?
     a. Theory of Planned Behavior
     b. Social Cognitive Theory
     c. Health Belief Model
     d. Socio-Ecological Model

16. What is motivational interviewing?
     a. An important part of the initial interview, it helps determine what motivates the client in his or her life.
     b. An important part of the initial interview when clients ask the trainer how he or she maintains an active lifestyle in an attempt to motivate the client.
     c. A helpful method of trainers to establish a points system to earn points for activity as a source of external motivation for a client.
     d. Acknowledging and working through a client's challenges concerning regular activity, stressing the fact that it is his or her choice to be active, while encouraging the change.

17. Women tend to have what kind of body fat distribution?
     a. Gynoid
     b. Android
     c. Abdominal
     d. Visceral

18. Which of the following lists the correct kilocalories per gram of the macronutrients?
     a. Carbohydrate 4 kcal, protein 4 kcal, alcohol 9 kcal, fat 9 kcal
     b. Carbohydrate 4 kcal, protein 4 kcal, alcohol 7 kcal, fat 9 kcal
     c. Carbohydrate 4 kcal, protein 9 kcal, alcohol 7 kcal, fat 9 kcal
     d. Carbohydrate 4 kcal, protein 4 kcal, alcohol 4 kcal, fat 9 kcal

19. Which of the following is FALSE regarding the female athlete triad?
     a. It can put an athlete at greater risk for fracture.
     b. Although it's called the female athlete triad, males can also have it.
     c. Females with the triad typically have infertility issues.
     d. It can increase risk of musculoskeletal injuries.

20. According to USDA recommendations, which of the following is not true?
     a. Eat at least half of your grains as whole grains
     b. Focus on low-fat and fat-free dairy over full fat
     c. Consume a variety of whole food (unprocessed and unrefined) vegetables and fruits
     d. Limit seafood intake

21. Optimal hydration is ideal, but what is the minimum recommended replacement rate for fluid lost during exercise?
     a. 8 oz. for every pound lost
     b. One cup for every pound lost
     c. One pint for every pound lost
     d. One quart for every pound lost

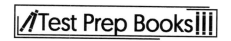

22. Which is NOT a component of the female athlete triad?
    a. Amenorrhea
    b. Overtraining
    c. Loss of bone density
    d. Disordered eating

23. What is the maximum amount of water as measured by percent body weight that can be lost before significant decline in performance and health occur?
    a. 1 to 3 percent
    b. 3 to 5 percent
    c. 5 to 8 percent
    d. 8 to 10 percent

24. You have been training Sarah for two years. Initially she was 120 pounds at 5'4" and now she is 101 pounds. She often gets weak and dizzy during workouts, and you notice she does the elliptical on her own over two hours per day. She also has become more withdrawn and never partakes in any of the meet-and-greet snack buffets at the fitness center anymore. While you can't be sure, you suspect she may be battling which of the following?
    a. Type 1 diabetes
    b. Anorexia nervosa
    c. Bulimia nervosa
    d. Type 2 diabetes

25. As a client's fitness level improves, what may become less important?
    a. Sources of external motivation
    b. Sources of internal motivation
    c. Setting S.M.A.R.T. goals
    d. Feedback

26. Which of the following is NOT within the scope of practice of a certified personal trainer?
    a. Stretching a client after a session
    b. Listening to a client's concerns about his stressful job
    c. Prescribing a home exercise program
    d. Making dietary recommendations for post-workout snacks

27. Karen wants to lose 20 pounds, which would put her BMI at 23 kg/m². She wants your recommendation for how much of a calorie deficit she should aim for with healthy weight loss. What do you recommend for overall health improvement and weight loss?
    a. Eat 500 to 1000 fewer kcal per day
    b. Eat 1000 to 1500 fewer kcal per day
    c. Eat 250 to 500 fewer kcal per day and expend 250 to 500 more kcal per day
    d. Eat 500 to 1000 fewer kcal per day and expend 500 to 1000 more kcal per day

28. A pregnant client is found unconscious and not breathing. You send someone to call 911 and the scene is safe. How would you proceed with CPR/AED?
    a. Wait for EMS. You cannot give CPR or use an AED on a pregnant woman
    b. Begin CPR and rescue breathing but do not use an AED on a pregnant woman
    c. Begin CPR, rescue breathing, and normal adult AED intervention
    d. Give two rescue breaths and use AED as normal but do not do CPR chest compressions on a pregnant woman

29. Which of the following terms means a stretch or tear to ligaments at a joint?
    a. Sprain
    b. Strain
    c. Fracture
    d. Dislocation

30. Which of the following is NOT an intrinsic risk factor for musculoskeletal injury?
    a. Training program too advanced
    b. Obesity
    c. Abnormal bony alignment
    d. Strength or flexibility imbalances

31. Concerning the health dangers of extreme fad diets, which of the following is true?
    a. They are a waste of money
    b. They can make the client feel like a failure
    c. They can decrease exercise performance
    d. They can cause severe dehydration

32. The cabbage soup diet is an example of which of the following?
    a. A fad diet
    b. An effective way to shed 10 pounds
    c. A weekend cleanse
    d. Carbo loading

33. Spondylolisthesis may present as which of the following?
    a. Shoulder pain
    b. Neck pain
    c. Knee pain
    d. Low back pain

34. Recommended body fat levels for men age thirty-five and older is best described as which of the following ranges?
    a. 5 to 13 percent
    b. 3 to 5 percent
    c. 10 to 25 percent
    d. 20 to 25 percent

Answer Key and Explanations

1. B: There are a variety of things the trainers can do to provide a positive, supportive training environment such as giving encouraging feedback and reinforcement that is frequent and timely. Trainers should help clients set SMART goals, identify sources of intrinsic and extrinsic motivational aids, help the client form a dependable support system, and identify and tackle barriers to adherence.

2. A: Depending on the individual client's comfort, preferences, and the content of what needs to be discussed, trainers can rely on a variety of communication methods such as email, phone, text messaging, and face-to-face conversations.

3. B: Kinesthetic learners learn best through movement, physical involvement, and experience. Trainers working with kinesthetic learners should demonstrate an exercise and then have the client try a simplified version of the movement such as completing an unweighted repetition of the exercise or moving through a partial range of motion. Before trying the full resistance or movement, these intermediate steps can demonstrate understanding while reducing injury risk. Auditory learners grasp information best through listening, so Choice D would be best for them. Visual learners learn through watching an observation, so Choice C would be best for these learners. Intellectual or cognitive learners would do well with reading about proper squat technique.

4. C: As mentioned in question three, visual learners ideally learn through observing, so Choice C would be best for these individuals.

5. C: When using active listening, trainers try to understand the underlying meaning of what a client is saying and then demonstrate this understanding by paraphrasing and then confirming comprehension. Choice C is a good example of active listening because the trainer hears that the client is looking to lose a little weight and get in better shape, and then confirms understanding by paraphrasing this back to the client in question form. Choices A, B, and D do not use active listening and may display lack of empathy, especially in the case of choice D, which comes across as somewhat harsh.

6. B: This is an example of supportive feedback, which is a means of encouraging the client, particularly during difficult parts of a workout. Evaluative feedback helps the client understand what parts of a particular movement he or she is mastering and to make improvements on incorrect movements or form during the learning process. Descriptive feedback is provided at the completion of a movement or workout in a concise fashion, providing a summary of what was observed and what can be improved or changed in subsequent efforts. Corrective feedback should be given to a client immediately, especially if something is unsafe.

7. A: This is an example of evaluative feedback, which is a means of encouraging the client during challenging parts of a workout. This type of feedback guides the client to make improvements with form or movements and fosters a greater understanding of what parts he or she is mastering in a given exercise or workout.

8. D: Obese. John's BMI is 30.1 kg/m^2 which puts him in the obese category (greater than 30 kg/m^2). The BMI categories are: Underweight = BMI of less than 18.5, Normal weight = 18.5 to 24.9, Overweight = 25 to 29.9, Obesity = BMI of 30 or greater.

9. D: Feedback should be timely and given as soon as possible after movement assessment while it is still fresh in the client's mind. Options B and C are incorrect because the trainer should give feedback more often than just after assessments or sporadically. Feedback provides motivation and when it is descriptive, corrective, or evaluative, it provides education and helps the client to improve. Option A is not necessarily wrong, but should just occur more than after every session, including after assessments as well as individual exercises within a given workout.

10. B: Programmatic barriers include not knowing how to structure a workout or what exercises to perform and in what way; previously attempting programs that were too hard, causing injury, frustration, or burnout; or programs that were too time-consuming, causing the client to feel like a failure. On the opposite end of the spectrum, programs that are not challenging enough can also cause boredom and lead to staleness, leading to program abandonment. By designing customized, appropriately challenging, and varied exercise programs, trainers can help keep clients engaged and improving towards their goals.

11. A: The Socio-Ecological Model addresses relationships and considers that behaviors, such as a client's motivation to exercise, are influenced by interpersonal relations in the surrounding environment, community, policy, and law. Using this model, trainers can improve program adherence by ensuring the client has a good social support system such as an exercise buddy and an environment conducive to exercise such as a gym in a convenient location or a recreational sports league close to work.

12. A: Goals that are not challenging enough have a tendency to cause the client's motivation to drop. Trainer should help clients set a mixture of both short-term and long-term goals. The risk of major relapses in healthy behaviors can be reduced by assuring clients that short lapses are inevitable and should not be considered failures, ensuring the social support system is positive and consistent, and making a list of possible causes of relapses and using the list to brainstorm solutions for when such issues arise.

13. A: There cannot really be too much intrinsic motivation and the more intrinsic motivation clients have, the more likely they are to continue with their healthy behavior.

14. D: Establishing a points system to win prizes after completing sessions each week is an example of a good external reward system for Tina. Because she is new to exercising, extrinsic rewards (factors outside of the exercise itself that help to support the desire to be physically active), may be especially important because the exercise itself is more painful and, because of discomfort and lack of fitness, less rewarding in and of itself.

Extrinsic rewards include things like a free T-shirt or iTunes gift card for workout music after completing a certain number of sessions. S.M.A.R.T. goals should be set as well, and reduced session fees may work. However, twenty sessions is a lot when a new client is struggling to get through each one. Neither of these choices is likely to be as good a motivating factor initially as the points system because they may feel intangible. Reminding her of the benefits of exercise and the risks of inactivity is an intrinsic reward and likely more motivating later on.

15. B: The Social Cognitive Theory states that behavioral change is influenced by the triad of interactions of the environment, personal factors, and behavior itself. Trainers can help clients develop self-regulatory strategies such as self-monitoring physical activity and setting personal goals and rewards, planning activity in advance, and having reasonable expectations. The trainer should help the client build self-efficacy.

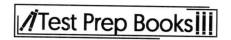

16. D: Motivational interviewing asks clients to reflect on what may happen if they do not change their current habits and weigh the pros and cons of activity and inactivity. It involves acknowledging and slowly working through a client's challenges concerning regular activity and stressing the fact that it is the individual's choice to be active.

17. A: Due to being estrogen dominant, females tend to have a gynoid, or pear-shaped distribution of body fat (accumulated more on the hips and thighs). Testosterone in higher concentrations causes an android or apple-shaped fat distribution in men, concentrating more body fat on the abdomen as visceral fat.

18. B: The energy in kcal for the macronutrients are as follows: carbohydrate 4 kcal, protein 4 kcal, alcohol 7 kcal, and fat 9 kcal.

19. B: The female athlete triad is a condition that only females experience. One of the cornerstones is amenorrhea, or cessation of menstrual cycle, which can cause infertility issues. While men can have disordered eating, they do not have the triad effect of the amenorrhea and its subsequent hormonal influence on reducing bone density. The female athlete triad can increase the risk of fracture and musculoskeletal injury, due to the loss of bone mass and the negative energy balance, which compromises recovery and healing.

20. D: The USDA encourages seafood consumption a minimum of twice per week, as well as making at least half of all grains whole grains, focusing on low-fat and fat-free dairy over full fat, and consuming a variety of whole food vegetables and fruits.

21. C: Optimal hydration is ideal, which would mean equal intake for excretion, but a minimum of one pint should be consumed for every pound lost during exercise, and then more can be consumed after exercise is over.

22. B: Overtraining is not directly part of the female athlete triad, although it may feed into some types of disordered eating. Amenorrhea, disordered eating, and loss of bone density are the three components of the triad.

23. B: Before experiencing significant performance-reducing dehydration, studies show that the body can experience a loss of about 3 to 5 percent of total mass in water. Beyond 5 percent, dehydration is too severe, and the person can suffer dangerous health and performance loss.

24. B: Sarah may be suffering from anorexia nervosa, an eating or body image disorder consisting of starvation and inadequate intake. It can lead to dizziness, and her compulsive cardio workouts are consistent with a desire to burn calories. Sarah seems to be avoiding eating as well.

25. A: As a client's fitness level improves, the act of exercising becomes less painful and more internally rewarding, so sources of external motivation may become less important. Intrinsic rewards are ones the client feels directly from the exercise itself and remain important long after goal achievement. They include things such as improved self-esteem or fitting into his or her favorite jeans. Intrinsically motivated clients, or those with self-determination, enjoy the process of the exercise itself, which tends to help them may maintain their health behaviors more easily than externally motivated clients, who exercise for the sake of achieving some sort of reward.

26. C: This was a tricky question. While providing home exercise programs is a common task for personal trainers, trainers must be careful not to "prescribe" anything, even workouts, because prescribing indicates medical or curative expertise, and that falls outside of the personal trainer's scope of practice. Trainers may create and provide home exercise programs. The other options are all valid too.

27. C: ACSM recommends a daily calorie deficit of 500 to 1000 kcal for those looking to lose weight, so options *A* or *C* are the first to be considered. The recommendation is that this deficit is achieved through increasing physical activity to raise energy expenditure and simultaneously reduce caloric intake. This dual-pronged approach has been shown to improve total health in addition to helping reduce weight, because physical activity is independently associated with greater health, while adding activity preserves lean body mass during a caloric deficit.

28. C: Certified personal trainers are required to act in cases of emergency and maintain CPR and AED certifications. A pregnant client receives CPR and AED the same as all other adult victims. In fact, it's even more important because two lives are on the line!

29. A: A sprain is a stretch or tear to ligaments at a joint while strains are tears or stretches to tendons and muscles. Fractures are cracks or breaks in bones or cartilage and dislocations occur when joint articulations become incongruous.

30. A: Extrinsic risk factors are those that influence injury risk outside of the individual such as training programming errors. Intrinsic risk factors are directly related to the individual and are typically physical in nature, such as obesity, abnormal bony alignment, or strength of flexibility imbalances.

31. D: One of the health dangers of extreme fad diets is severe dehydration. Wasting money, causing the client to feel like a failure, and decreased exercise performance can be considered cons of fad diets, but not necessarily "health dangers" in the way that dehydration can be.

32. A: The cabbage soup diet is an example of a fad diet. Fad diets are ones that are popularized in the media and may make unreasonable promises or be dangerous, too limiting, or not possible or healthy to continue long term.

33. D: Spondylolisthesis is a fracture in the pars interarticularis of the spine and presents as low back pain. It is especially prevalent in adolescent athletes in sports requiring spinal extension such as gymnastics and weightlifting.

34. C: Recommended body fat levels for men age thirty-five and older is 10 to 25 percent.

Legal & Professional Responsibilities

Reputable Referral Sources

Trainers should ensure referrals to other professionals are reputable and competent. Professionals should carry current certification or licensure from industry leaders. When networking with such professionals, trainers should be aware that referrals can work both ways, and that through professional and positive relationships with other local clinicians, they may get referrals back for exercise programming. It is prudent to either read reviews or speak to a trusted individual or practice about any new provider before adding him or her to a referral list. In the personal training industry alone, there are an increasing number of uncertified trainers or those with overnight "certifications" from websites that do not necessarily ensure competency.

Scope of Practice

Certified Personal Trainers are involved in the education, motivation, assessment, and training of clients toward health and fitness goals and should refer clients to other health professionals when working with issues outside of this scope of practice. It is imperative that trainers respect the boundaries of their scope of practice and do not attempt to diagnose, treat, counsel, or prescribe, or they may be subjected to liability and malpractice. While "exercise is medicine" is a common idea and has truths to it, trainers should refrain from using terms like "exercise prescription" or "this exercise will treat your condition," and instead refer to the "exercise program." While clients may rely heavily on the advice and expertise of trainers, often asking questions outside of a trainer's scope of practice, the trainer can educate on topics within his or her scope. However, they must refer to appropriate sources for all else.

Professional Communication Health Professionals

Trainers are allied health professionals, and as such, are part of the medical community. They need to be able to communicate effectively with physicians and other health professionals on an ongoing basis to follow up on client referrals and progress using adherence to HIPAA and confidentiality guidelines. Trainers should be mindful to use proper medical and anatomical terminology so they do not lose credibility and are effective communicators.

Identifying Individuals Requiring Referrals

Trainers should form a network of various types of healthcare providers such as physicians, physical therapists, mental health professionals, chiropractors, and nutritionists in order to provide clients with comprehensive, reputable care. Appropriate referrals minimize liability by ensuring the trainer acts only within his or her scope of practice. It also maximizes program effectiveness by addressing the many concerns and challenges faced by clients, which may otherwise prevent full exercise participation and goal achievement.

Clients with injuries may need to see their physician, an orthopedist, or physical therapists. Clients with weight issues or dietary concerns may benefit from a referral to a dietician or weight management specialist. Psychological and social services may be necessary for other clients. Trainers should not only identify the appropriate professional, but help facilitate the introduction in a respectful and positive manner.

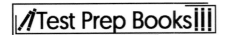

Comprehensive Risk Management Program

Risk management reduces liability for trainers, but also raises the standard of care for clients and keeps their safety and health in the forefront. Clients should not only be properly stratified and have all necessary medical forms, consent, and waivers signed and on file, but they should also be educated on medical, environmental, and facility emergency procedures. All emergency procedures should be documented in written form, rehearsed and posted under each phone. An injury prevention program such as RICES (rest, ice, compression, elevation, stabilization) should be used.

CPR and AED

Trainers must be trained in basic life support, and keep current CPR and AED (automated external defibrillator) certification and be prepared to respond with emergency cardiac care in cases of myocardial infarction (MI) or sudden cardiac arrest (SCA). It is beneficial if the facility has emergency oxygen and the trainer is versed in administering it during cases of suspected mild to moderate MI, while waiting for emergency medical personnel to arrive on scene. Failure to keep current CPR and AED certification is a liability risk for trainers and may also void personal training certification status.

Emergency Procedures

Emergency procedures should be written and practiced every three months by all involved staff. It is important to keep emergency equipment up to date and documented as such, have established telephone procedures, required equipment, emergency response contacts, map of emergency exits and fire extinguishers, and specific documented responsibilities that are rehearsed by staff members. Trainers should explain the emergency procedures to each new client and remind him or her periodically or if changes are made.

Providing a Safe Exercise Setting

Precautions employed in the exercise setting can improve client safety. Trainers should ensure that routine maintenance is performed and documented on all equipment by trained professionals and that equipment is being used in the proper way. The surface floor should be tidy and free from potential tripping hazards. If exercising outside, trainers should heed warning to environmental conditions such as excessive heat, humidity, storms, cold, and wind, and terminate sessions or relocate indoors if any threats exist.

Spotting

Once a trainer is comfortable with the client's understanding of an exercise, the client should be tasked with performing the exercise as modeled. While the client is engaging in the exercise, a trainer should remain focused on the client's form and technique, supporting and assisting to ensure that injury does not occur. Spotting clients by being in front, behind, or beside them throughout the performance not only reassures the client that the exercise is being performed correctly and without risk, but also enables the trainer to be in position to relieve the client of the weight being used, or to help them disengage from the posture of the exercise should it become uncomfortable. During spotting, trainers should use a wide stance, slight bend in the knee, and have their hands on or close to the weights.

Musculoskeletal Injuries Terms

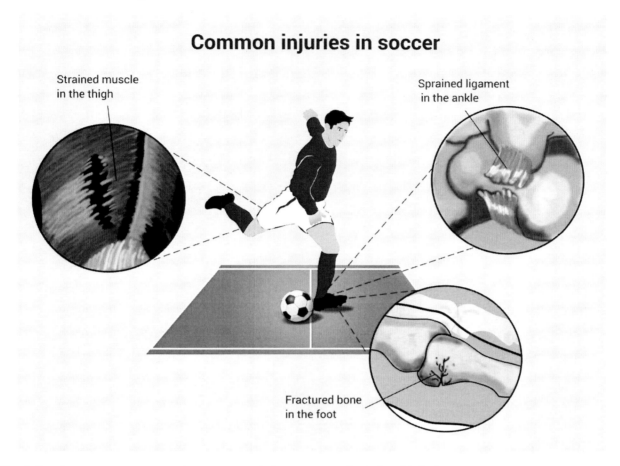

Common injuries in soccer

Strained muscle in the thigh

Sprained ligament in the ankle

Fractured bone in the foot

The following are some general terms pertaining to musculoskeletal injuries:

- Shin splints: inflammatory overuse injury of the medial shin, often from running

- Sprain: stretch or tear to ligaments at a joint

- Strain: damage to tendons or muscles at the tendinous junction

- Bursitis: inflammation of bursae, fluid-filled sacs that lubricate and cushion joints or subcutaneous tissue

- Fracture: a break or crack in bone or cartilage

- Tendonitis: tendon inflammation often from overuse injury

- Patellar-femoral pain syndrome: also called "Runner's knee," pain in the patella tendon, which is the insertion point for the quadriceps muscles just below the kneecap, often from jumping or improper squatting or improper tracking of the patella

- Low back pain: common "catch-all" complaint, can be from disc dysfunction, muscle strain, spinal stenosis of the lumbar spine, spondylolisthesis and other causes

- Plantar fasciitis: pain in the heel/sole of the foot, worse in the morning, from inflammation of the plantar fascia – a band of tissue on the sole and arch of the foot

Contraindicated Exercises

Many stretches and exercises once thought to be healthy are actually dangerous and can lead to injury. Some examples include:

- Straight-leg sit-ups: strains lower back muscles and hyperextends the iliopsoas, targeting hip flexors instead of abdominals

- Cervical and lumbar hyperextensions: can cause injury to ligaments, discs, and muscles in the neck and back

- Deep full squats: extreme flexion causes knee ligaments and cartilage to become overstressed

- Double leg raises: arches the low back and puts strain on low back muscles and ligaments

- Hurdler's stretch: one leg out straight and the other bent behind the body can cause groin pull, hip discomfort (femur in extreme rotation), injure knee cartilage, and overstretch the medial collateral ligament.

- Standing toe-touches: uses ballistic movement that can cause injury; with knees locked, puts undue stress on the lumbar spine

Responsibilities to Perform Emergency Procedures

Trainers are responsible and held liable for appropriately and safely caring for clients under their watch during emergency situations, both with the client directly and at the fitness facility. Trainers must be knowledgeable of and prepared to perform current emergency action plans and ensure client safety as much as possible.

Injury Risk Factors

Musculoskeletal injuries are unfortunately a fairly common adverse effect of exercise, cited to be about two to three injuries per participant per year. There are intrinsic and extrinsic risk factors that interact and predispose a client to injury, but the most common causes are poor baseline fitness, overtraining, improper biomechanics, and improper training techniques. Other intrinsic risk factors are history of previous injury or musculoskeletal disease, obesity, abnormal bony alignment, strength or flexibility imbalances, or joint or ligamentous laxity. Extrinsic factors are type (impact) and speed of movement, improper footwear or surface, fatigue, or environmental conditions. Trainers should work to reduce modifiable risk factors by maintaining safe equipment and training environments, appropriately progressing new clients, giving adequate rest, and mixing modalities and exercises to build a balanced, strong body and prevent overtraining.

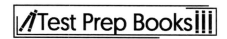

Initial Management of Various Complications

While medical clearance helps prevent complications during exercise, trainers need to be prepared to administer help should issues such as the following arise:

Open wounds: Trainer must employ universal precautions (such as latex gloves) and wash hands immediately after. Use soap and water to clean minor wounds, then cover with germicide cream and a sterile bandage. Use a flat hand and fingers to apply pressure and control the bleeding in major wounds and elevate above client's heart as long as no fracture is suspected. Call EMS and place pressure over the brachial or femoral artery if bleeding is not slowing for upper or lower extremity injuries, respectively.

Musculoskeletal injuries: Use RICES (rest, ice, compression, elevation, and stabilization) as long as no fracture is suspected.

Cardiovascular/pulmonary complications (asthma attack, angina): Stop exercise immediately when signs or symptoms appear such as: pain in the chest, head, neck, jaw, or arms, heart palpitations, dizziness or syncope, intermittent claudication, hyperventilation or unusual shortness of breath, an inability to speak. Emergency medical personnel should be called immediately if symptoms persist once exercise is stopped and client is supine, if possible. Client should see a physician prior to resuming exercise, and the trainer should speak to the physician.

Metabolic disorders (hypo- or hyperglycemia): Stop exercise immediately and test blood sugar if a glucometer is available. Administer glucose in the form of food or drink if blood sugar is low. Signs include: shakiness, weakness, abnormal sweating, mouth or finger tingling, visual disturbances, confusion, and seizures. Clients with known metabolic disease should speak with physicians prior to exercise programs or when programming changes about insulin and glucose needs before, during, and after exercise and carry supplies with them.

Basic First-Aid
It is beneficial for trainers to get basic first-aid certification for proper knowledge and confidence of applying treatment to clients. Even in the absence of certification, trainers should be prepared to administer basic first-aid to clients during sessions in case injuries occur such as the following:

- Strains/sprains: Use RICES: ice for twenty to thirty minutes every two hours, elevate above the heart if possible, and use elastic wrap to apply compression for the first twenty-four to seventy-two hours.

- Fractures: Call EMS and, if possible, do not move client; calm and reassure them and provide an ice pack. Splints should not be used unless the client must be moved, in which case a proper splinting technique must be employed. Monitor for signs of shock, internal bleeding, or other emergencies.

- Exercise intolerance such as dizziness, syncope, and heat injury: Stop exercise immediately and try to get client supine. Provide water or sports drink if available. With suspected heat injuries, move client to shade or cooler environment, remove excess clothing, and apply cool water cloths on wrists, neck, and behind knees.

Equipment Service and Maintenance

Daily inspection of equipment and routine maintenance by trained professionals in accordance to manufacturer's guidelines should be documented and conducted to decrease risk of injury and liability. Cables and bands should be checked for thinning or fraying prior to each use, and belts and safety stops on treadmills should be evaluated for wear and function. Weights should be racked and loose equipment put back and stored away after use to prevent trips and falls. Equipment and mats should be cleaned between clients with antibacterial wash to avoid the spread of germs. Safety equipment such as AEDs and fire extinguishers should be checked monthly and its proper function should be documented. Malfunctioning equipment such as broken bands should be removed from the floor if possible or clearly marked with an "Out of Order" sign if not mobile.

Safety Policies and Procedures

Having comprehensive, well-thought-out and regularly rehearsed safety procedures decreases risk of unsafe behaviors, injury, and resultant liability. The absence of creating safety policies, training staff and clients in their use, and posting clear explanations of them (such as what to do in case of fire or power outage) in readily available places can result in negligence and legal responsibility on the part of the facility for any incurred injuries. Staff and clients should receive printed copies of all safety procedures, listen to a thorough explanation, rehearse them, and ask any questions for clarification. Incident reports should be completed and reviewed for every injury or safety issue that arises, looking for trends and better solutions for ongoing safety improvements.

Emergency Action Plan Components

Emergency plans should be written, explained orally, and practiced by staff and clients. Copies should be posted under each phone and distributed to staff and clients. As revisions are made, they should be explained and rehearsed. Emergency action plans should be comprehensive, clear, and concise and include things such as:

- Clearly marked exits with illuminated signs
- Fire extinguishers and a fire emergency safety plan, and emergency evacuation or shelter plans posted under each phone for things like floods, storms, and tornadoes
- Clearly delineated staff responsibilities
- Emergency Medical Services (EMS) contact activated on phones
- First aid kit, AED, latex gloves, blood pressure kit and stethoscope, CPR masks, etc.

Effectively Communicating Emergency Procedures

Trainers should effectively communicate with staff and clients all salient information about medical, environmental, and facility emergency policies procedures. All emergency procedures should be documented in written form, rehearsed and posted under each phone.

Demonstrating Emergency Procedures During Testing

Staff and supervising physicians should be aware of all emergency procedures during testing and training. Clients should be instructed how to stop the test at any moment should the need or desire arise. Emergency stop switches and buttons, such as those on treadmills, should always be engaged, and clients should be instructed on their use during testing and training.

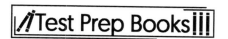

Assisting, Spotting, and Monitoring Clients Safely

The safety of clients during exercise testing and training is of utmost importance. It is the trainer's responsibility to optimize safety. Trainers must be diligent in observing, assisting, and correctly spotting clients during exercise. They should repeatedly demonstrate proper form and technique, providing detailed descriptions of the exercise's goals and common mistakes that pose risk of injury. Spotting and consistently providing verbal and nonverbal cues will help to ensure that the client masters the techniques and performance of exercises.

To ensure a client's safety and their ability to use equipment, the trainer must provide a thorough demonstration and carefully observe the client's performance of each exercise. Not only will this maximize the physiologic benefits and reduce risk of injury, but it will also help to improve the client's ability to master technique and form, allowing for the implementation of increasingly more challenging exercises.

ACSM's Code of Ethics

To promote safety and reduce liability risk, trainers should practice in a professional manner within the Scope of Practice of Certified Personal Trainers and adhere to ACSM's Code of Ethics. ACSM's Code of Ethics is a source of guidelines and expectations about ethical practices and responsibilities for all certified professionals and disciplinary actions if the codes are not met. The full Code of Ethics can be found at: certification.acsm.org/faq28-codeofethics.

Appropriate Work Attire

Personal trainers should be dressed professionally at all times. Clothing should be clean and modest, such as collared shirts, proper footwear, and athletic pants or shorts that are not overly tight or revealing. Trainers should remember to always demonstrate empathy and compassion, and remember that in addition to delivering sound programming and health and fitness advice, they are also in the customer service business. Clients should be treated with respect, addressed formally, and given undivided attention during sessions.

Conducting Activities within the Scope of Practice

ACSM trainers develop and implement individualized programming to clients based on sound exercise science principles. Under the scope of practice, trainers lead and demonstrate safe and effective exercise methods, write appropriate program recommendations, and motivate clients to begin and maintain healthy behaviors. ACSM trainers should always act professionally and within this scope of practice.

Professional Liability and Negligence

- Personal injury liability insurance protects against libel, slander, and invasion of privacy.

- Professional liability insurance protects against injuries caused by services or negligence.

- Commercial liability insurance covers individuals and the business against incidents and accidents that occurred at the facility and must be purchased by trainers who own their own studios.

- Negligence is a failure to perform at the accepted standard (due care), while gross negligence is to do so willingly. In addition to carrying the necessary liability insurance, trainers can help defend against negligence claims by documenting all services daily and performing to the highest industry standards.

Legal Risk-Management Techniques

To reduce risk of legal issues, certified personal trainers should respect and always work within the boundaries of their scope of practice. Diagnosing or treating medical issues and injuries or prescribing diets are not functions of a personal trainer and must be correctly referred to the appropriately licensed healthcare professional. Certification requirements, medical clearances, signed informed consents, and proper personal injury and professional liability insurance should always be maintained and up-to-date. Trainers should always employ their best judgment and a scientific approach to exercise testing and programming, being mindful of each client's ability level and current health to avoid risky exercises. They also should avoid making significant leaps in intensity or skill level, which may injure clients. If home exercises or unsupervised sessions are expected of clients, trainers should fully explain and demonstrate exactly how to complete such tasks.

Equipment Maintenance to Decrease Risk

As mentioned, to decrease the risk of injury and liability, daily inspection of equipment and routine maintenance by trained professionals in accordance to manufacturer's guidelines should be documented and conducted. Cables and bands should be checked for thinning or fraying prior to each use, and belts and safety stops on treadmills should be evaluated for wear and function. Weights should be racked and loose equipment put back and stored away after use to prevent trips and falls. Equipment and mats should be cleaned between clients with antibacterial wash to avoid the spread of germs. Safety equipment such as AEDs and fire extinguishers should be checked monthly and its proper function should be documented. Malfunctioning equipment such as broken bands should be removed from the floor if possible or clearly marked with an "Out of Order" sign if not mobile.

Floors also require regular cleaning. Non-absorbent surfaces should be mopped, wooden platforms should be monitored for cracks, and regular dusting should remove and prevent grime buildup; these actions will help keep the floor free of obstacles and prevent slips and falls.

Copyright Laws

Trainers looking to protect their own intellectual property can apply for protection under United States Copyright Laws by going to Copyright.gov. This website, maintained by the United States Copyright Office, also contains information, laws, and policies about copyrighting material and using protected material. While no single global international copyright exists, trainers desiring copyright protection for their work in a particular country should determine the extent of protection available to works of foreign authors in that specific country.

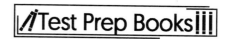

Respecting Copyrights

National and international copyright laws should be obeyed to protect original work, intellectual property, and educational resources and to legally use media and information published by others without consequence.

Documentation of Non-Original Work

All non-original work (videos, articles, images, etc.) must be properly cited and attributed to its creator to prevent copyright infringements and plagiarism.

Safeguard Client Confidentiality

All sensitive and identifying client information should be safely stored and kept confidential and private, unless clients formally waive these privacy rights in writing or if this information must be accessed in emergency situations.

Systems for Maintaining Client Confidentiality

Trainers and facilities should have systems in place to ensure sensitive client information is kept confidential. Hard copy files should be locked in file cabinets, with key accessibility for intended audiences only. When trainers wish to communicate about a client with a physician, healthcare professional, other trainer, or a client's family member, they must obtain written and signed permission from the client and add this form, along with a timeframe beyond which this authorization is no longer valid, to the chart.

Importance of Client Privacy

Client files should be kept private to protect clients from identity or credit card theft, respect medical laws of confidentiality, and protect the trainer from legal liability by breaching these privacy laws.

FERPA and HIPAA Laws

The Family Educational Rights and Privacy Act (FERPA) relates mainly to protected information involving education, particularly in school settings. The Health Insurance Portability and Accountability Act (HIPAA) of 1996 defines individually identifiable health information such as demographics, prior and current health history, social security number, etc. The purpose of these laws is to protect sensitive client information and ensure this identifiable and personal information is kept only for the intended professionals. Trainers and fitness facilities must be sure to comply with these laws and lock up and otherwise encrypt all client files.

Rapid Access to Client Information

A client's file with all health, demographics, prior workouts, and emergency contact information should be with the trainer during testing and training sessions with that client. Should an emergency arise, trainers and staff need to have quick and easy access to pertinent information on the client such as emergency contact numbers, physician's name and number, and allergies. To abide by the laws of confidentiality and patient privacy, trainers should be sure to keep this file safely out of the hands of other people during sessions. If the trainer stores this information digitally, a computer or tablet should be turned on and accessed in the event of an emergency.

Practice Questions

1. Which of the following is within the scope of practice of a certified personal trainer?
   a. Diagnosing a meniscal tear
   b. Making a customized nutrition plan for a client
   c. Giving a cross-friction massage for scar tissue
   d. Teaching the client exercises to do during work travel assignments

2. Benefits of spotting a client during exercise include all EXCEPT which of the following?
   a. Ensuring the client is using correct form
   b. Demonstrating good spotting form so the client can help you
   c. Making sure the client and surrounding clients are safe
   d. Staying more actively engaged as the trainer

3. Which of the following defines individually identifiable health information such as demographics, prior and current health history, social security number, etc.?
   a. Health Insurance Portability and Accountability Act (HIPAA)
   b. Health Insurance Portability and Privacy Act (HIPPA)
   c. Family Exercise Rights and Privacy Act (FERPA)
   d. Family Educational Rights and Privacy Act (FERPA)

4. To reduce liability risk, trainers should do all EXCEPT which of the following?
   a. Adhere to ACSM risk stratification and guidelines for clearance and medical supervision
   b. Rehearse emergency action plans and maintain CPR certification
   c. Abide by the ACSM Scope of Practice for certified personal trainers and adhere to the Code of Ethics
   d. Model healthy lifestyle and behavior choices

5. To be stratified as low risk, a client must meet which of the following conditions?
   I. Males less than forty-five years of age or females less than fifty-five years
   II. Asymptomatic
   III. Have no risk factors for cardiovascular or pulmonary disease
   IV. Have one risk factor for cardiovascular or pulmonary disease

   a. I and III only
   b. II and III only
   c. I, II, and III
   d. I, II, and IV

6. Ethan is a 21-year-old college student who plays on the baseball team. He is coming to you for strengthening. He is 70 inches tall and weighs 160 pounds. He doesn't smoke and both parents are healthy. He was diagnosed with Type 1 diabetes at age 8, but his blood glucose is normal with insulin injections. His blood pressure is 105/68 mmHg and his total cholesterol is 170 mg/dL. He reports no symptoms and can train after practice and on weekends. In what risk category is Ethan?
   a. No risk
   b. Low risk
   c. Moderate risk
   d. High risk

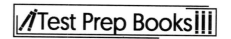

7. Kathleen is a 23-year-old client who lives with both parents. She is 64 inches tall and weighs 128 pounds. Her blood pressure today is 116/75 mmHg and her total cholesterol is 170 mg/dL, with LDL at 120 and blood glucose at 82 mg/dL. She dances or plays volleyball most days of the week and smokes, but only on the weekends with friends. How many risk factors for CAD does Kathleen have?
   a. Zero
   b. One
   c. Two
   d. Three

8. Janice is a 58-year-old sedentary female coming to you to "get in shape," since she has "not worked out since college." She is 180 pounds and 5'4." She has no personal history of heart disease and quit smoking 3 years ago, but her mother had a myocardial infarction (MI) at the age of 66. Janice's blood pressure is consistently 135/85 mmHg, total cholesterol is 180 mg/dL, with an HDL level of 30 mg/dL, and fasting blood glucose is 90 mg/dL.
How many risk factors for CAD does Janice have?
   a. Two
   b. Three
   c. Four
   d. Five

9. Which of the following statements is true about medical clearance prior to participating in an exercise training program?
   a. All clients need medical clearance from a physician prior to participation in an exercise training program.
   b. Only clients with diagnosed cardiovascular, respiratory, or metabolic diseases need clearance prior to participation.
   c. Children, adolescents, men less than forty-five years, and women less than fifty-five years who do not have CAD risk factors or symptoms, known disease, and who did not answer "yes" to any questions on the PAR-Q do not need clearance.
   d. Children, adolescents, men less than fifty years, and women less than fifty-five years who do not have CAD risk factors or symptoms, known disease, and who did not answer "yes" to any questions on the PAR-Q do not need clearance.

10. When a certified personal trainer fails to perform what is typically considered to be a standard practice of care, it may be deemed to be which of the following?
   a. Negligence
   b. Malpractice
   c. Liability
   d. Scope of Practice

11. If a piece of moveable equipment is broken, what should you do?
   a. Attach an "Out of Order" sign
   b. Let it be but avoid using it in a workout
   c. Remove it from the floor
   d. Unplug it

12. What pieces of equipment should be evaluated prior to every single use?

       I. Medicine balls

       II. Exercise bands

       III. Cables on weight machines

       IV. Emergency stop buttons on cardio equipment

    a. All of the above

    b. I, III, IV

    c. II, III, IV

    d. III, IV

13. Which of the following could breach the safety of privacy for paper client files?

    a. Locking up paper files

    b. Scanning and making digital copies for the facility computer

    c. Carrying the paper file on your clipboard during sessions and keeping it on your person at all times

    d. Making sure keys are only given to authorized individuals

14. When can private, personal identifying information from a client's file be accessed without permission?

    a. When a new trainer fills in

    b. When the client is having a medical emergency

    c. When the spouse needs to access information

    d. When sending in taxes so the IRS can get a copy

15. Which of the following are contraindicated exercises?

    a. Straight-leg sit-ups, double leg raises, standing toe-touches, deep squats

    b. Straight-leg sit-ups, side planks, standing toe-touches, deep squats

    c. Abdominal crunches, double leg raises, standing toe-touches, deep squats

    d. Abdominal crunches, side planks, standing toe-touches, deep squats

16. How would you treat a minor open wound?

    a. Employ universal precautions (such as latex gloves) and wash hands immediately after. Use soap and water to clean the wound, then leave open to air out.

    b. Employ universal precautions (such as latex gloves) and wash hands immediately after. Use a germicide cream and cover with a sterile bandage.

    c. Employ universal precautions (such as latex gloves) and wash hands immediately after. Use soap and water to clean the wound, then cover with germicide cream and a sterile bandage.

    d. Employ universal precautions (such as latex gloves) and wash hands immediately after. Use a flat hand and fingers to apply pressure and control the bleeding in minor wounds and elevate it above the client's heart as long as no fracture is suspected.

17. Shakiness, weakness, abnormal sweating, mouth or finger tingling, visual disturbances, confusion, and seizures can be signs of what?

    a. Hyperglycemia

    b. Hypoglycemia

    c. Overtraining

    d. Sudden cardiac arrest

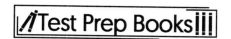

18. How often should emergency procedures should be reviewed and rehearsed?
    a. Every month
    b. Every week
    c. Every three months
    d. Twice per year

19. RICES for acute injury treatment stands for?
    a. Rest, Ice, Compression, Elevation, Stabilization
    b. Rest, Ice, Compression, Elevation, Splint
    c. Rest, Injury, Compression, Elevation, Splint
    d. Rest, Injury, Compression, Elevation, Stabilization

Answer Key and Explanations

1. D: Teaching the client exercises to do during work travel assignments helps avoid relapses in healthy behaviors and is prudent for certified personal trainers to do to help clients develop self-efficacy and an exercise habit, despite the barrier of travel. Customized nutrition plans should be from registered dieticians or nutritionists; licensed massage therapists should provide therapeutic massage; and diagnosing meniscal tears is the role of a physician.

2. B: Spotting clients while lifting weights and assisting clients with all types of equipment and exercises helps monitor their form and provides an effort to reduce injury risk and maximize training benefit. It helps prevent weights from dropping and rolling, which can distract and injure others in the vicinity. It is not for the trainer's personal workout benefit.

3. A: Health Insurance Portability and Accountability Act (HIPAA) defines individually identifiable health information such as demographics, prior and current health history, social security number, etc. FERPA is the Family Educational Rights and Privacy Act, and it relates mainly to protected information about education, particularly in school settings.

4. D: While modeling a healthy lifestyle is important, it does not reduce liability risk for trainers. Trainers should be mindful to adhere to ACSM risk stratification and guidelines for clearance and medical supervision, rehearse emergency action plans, maintain CPR certification, abide by the ACSM Scope of Practice for certified personal trainers and adhere to the Code of Ethics.

5. D: A client is low risk if they have one or fewer risk factors, but he or she should still be asymptomatic, and less than the age of forty-five or fifty-five for men and women, respectively. Condition III has no risk factors, but the client can have up to one, so all of the other choices are invalid.

6. D: Ethan is high risk because he has a known metabolic disease – the Type 1 diabetes. The other risk factors do not factor into his stratification because having the disease automatically makes him high risk.

7. B: Kathleen has one risk factor – smoking. Her BMI is normal, she has no known family medical history, healthy blood pressure and blood work, and she is active.

8. C: Janice has the following four risk factors: obesity (her BMI at 30.9 is greater than 30 kg/m^2), low HDL (<40 mg/dL), physical inactivity, and age > 55. Smoking is not a risk factor, since she quit more than six months ago. Her blood pressure and fasting glucose are normal. Although her mother died of an MI, this does not count as a risk factor at age 66.

9. C: Clients who are apparently healthy are not required to get medical clearance prior to starting an exercise program. This includes children, adolescents, men less than forty-five years, and women less than fifty-five years who do not have CAD risk factors or symptoms, known disease, and who did not answer "yes" to any questions on the PAR-Q. *A* and *B* are not correct, and *D* provides too high of an age cutoff for "apparently healthy males."

10. A: When a certified personal trainer fails to perform what is typically considered to be a standard practice of care, it may be deemed to be negligence.

11. C: Because it was specified that the piece of broken equipment was movable, it should be picked up and removed from the floor so that it is not accidentally used, possibly leading to injury. Failing to do so

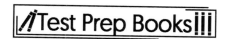

would be an example of negligence, and gross negligence if the trainer was aware of the issue and left it there anyway. An "Out of Order" sign could be used for treadmills or large equipment that could not be easily removed, but it is safer to take the piece off the floor so the sign is not accidentally removed and the broken equipment used.

12. C: Medicine balls should be checked weekly or so for cracks, which can cause sand to leak. Unless they are old or used a lot, medicine balls do not need to be checked prior to every use. More importantly, even if they do have sand leaks, they should not injure a client when they are starting to fall apart. Exercise bands routinely thin and can snap, and cables often fray, both of which can be very dangerous. Emergency stop buttons on cardio equipment should also be checked prior to usage.

13. B: Scanning and making digital copies of client files for the facility computer could breach privacy unless the files are password-protected.

14. B: A client's file with all health, demographics, prior workouts, and emergency contact information should be with the trainer during testing and training sessions with that client. Should an emergency arise, trainers and staff need to have quick and easy access to pertinent information. Trainers need to obtain written and signed permission for other distribution of the file.

15. A: Straight-leg sit-ups, double leg raises, standing toe-touches, and deep squats are contraindicated because the risk-to-benefit ratio is poor. They are likely to cause injury, and the same muscles can be exercised more safely. With proper form, abdominal crunches and side planks are safe.

16. C: Universal precautions (such as latex gloves), washing the wound with soap and water, then covering it with germicide cream and a sterile bandage is the basic treatment for all minor wounds. Trainers assisting clients with minor wounds should always wash their hands immediately after treatment, even with the use of latex gloves. To control the bleeding in major wounds, use a flat hand and fingers to apply pressure, then elevate the affected body part above the client's heart as long as no fracture is suspected. Trainers should call EMS and place pressure over the brachial or femoral artery if bleeding is not slowing for upper or lower extremity injuries, respectively.

17. B: Signs of hypoglycemia include shakiness, weakness, abnormal sweating, mouth or finger tingling, visual disturbances, confusion, and seizures. If such symptoms occur, the trainer should stop exercise immediately and use a glucometer to test blood sugar, if possible. If blood sugar is low, trainers should administer glucose in the form of food or drink.

18. C: To ensure understanding and preparedness, emergency procedures should be reviewed and rehearsed by involved staff at least quarterly (every three months).

19. A: Acute injury treatment should employ RICES: Rest, Ice, Compression, Elevation, Stabilization.

Dear ACSM Test Taker,

We would like to start by thanking you for purchasing this study guide for your ACSM exam. We hope that we exceeded your expectations.

Our goal in creating this study guide was to cover all of the topics that you will see on the test. We also strove to make our practice questions as similar as possible to what you will encounter on test day. With that being said, if you found something that you feel was not up to your standards, please send us an email and let us know.

We would also like to let you know about other books in our catalog that may interest you.

ACE	amazon.com/dp/1628457740
CSCS	amazon.com/dp/1637752148
NASM	amazon.com/dp/1628457996

We have study guides in a wide variety of fields. If the one you are looking for isn't listed above, then try searching for it on Amazon or send us an email.

Thanks Again and Happy Testing!
Product Development Team
info@studyguideteam.com

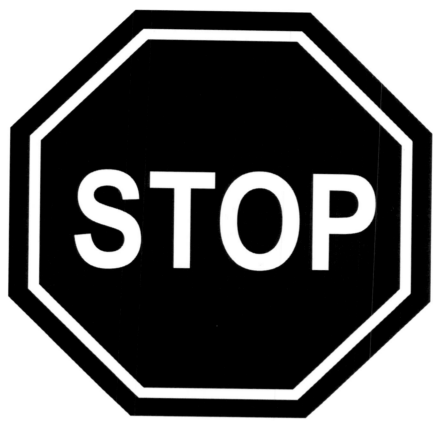

FREE Test Taking Tips DVD Offer

To help us better serve you, we have developed a Test Taking Tips DVD that we would like to give you for FREE. **This DVD covers world-class test taking tips that you can use to be even more successful when you are taking your test.**

All that we ask is that you email us your feedback about your study guide. Please let us know what you thought about it – whether that is good, bad or indifferent.

To get your **FREE Test Taking Tips DVD**, email freedvd@studyguideteam.com with "FREE DVD" in the subject line and the following information in the body of the email:

a. The title of your study guide.

b. Your product rating on a scale of 1-5, with 5 being the highest rating.

c. Your feedback about the study guide. What did you think of it?

d. Your full name and shipping address to send your free DVD.

If you have any questions or concerns, please don't hesitate to contact us at freedvd@studyguideteam.com.

Thanks again!

Made in United States
North Haven, CT
16 March 2023

34105243R00074